THE BRUISING APOTHECARY

IMAGES OF PHARMACY
AND
MEDICINE IN CARICATURE

Prints and Drawings in the Collection of the Museum of the Royal
Pharmaceutical Society of Great Britain

Kate Arnold-Forster
Nigel Tallis

London
THE PHARMACEUTICAL PRESS
1989

All photography by Rod Tidnam.

Cover Illustration : The bruising Apothecary – paratus operi – (catalogue no. 15).

Printed by BAS Printers Limited, Over Wallop, Hampshire.

CONTENTS

PREFACE AND ACKNOWLEDGMENTS

This catalogue has been prepared to provide an introduction to the subject of pharmacy and medicine in caricature, based on the collection of the Museum of the Royal Pharmaceutical Society of Great Britain. It is the first publication of its kind to be produced on the Society's Museum so it is hoped that it will stimulate interest in the collection, as well as the specialist field it covers.

Unlike more formal art forms, there is a unique and immediate quality to the art of caricature arising from its concern with contemporary social and political issues. The attitudes and events, and even the comic or satiric values, that affect the caricaturist are normally those of direct relevance to the audience they seek for their work. This is as true of the sketches of 18th century aristocratic amateurs as for the mass appeal of tabloid newspaper cartoons of the present. Thus these images, especially those reproduced and widely distributed as individual prints or in books, journals and periodicals, are an important, though subtle source of historical evidence on popular ideas of medicine and pharmacy and one that deserves further consideration.

In recent years, the interpretation of documentary records has greatly increased our knowledge of pharmaceutical and medical history but comparitively little attention has yet been paid to the examination of alternative historical records. A catalogue of a collection of this size, covering such an extensive subject area, cannot hope to make more than a modest contribution to the art historical study of this topic, but it may bring renewed consideration to more specific issues concerning the way medicine and pharmacy were seen in the past.

Many have helped in the preparation of this catalogue which has been made possible by recent work undertaken on the Museum documentation. In particular we are grateful for the support of the Area Museums Service for South-Eastern England; the considerable efforts of Susan Barber and Stella Mason; for the advice of Ralph Hyde, William Schupbach, Doris Jones and Sydney Holloway and, above all, for the assistance of our colleagues, particularly Pamela North and Mairead Mackenzie, at the Royal Pharmaceutical Society of Great Britain.

Kate Arnold-Forster
Nigel Tallis

INTRODUCTION

The Art of Caricature

The word caricature is derived from the Italian 'caricare', to overload. By exaggerating features of physiognomy the artist creates an image to convey a comic effect. The humorous use of distortion has been adopted throughout many forms of artistic representation but its use to identify particular characteristics with specific individuals was only established by the late Renaissance. The term was first adopted by the Bolognese draughtsman, Annibale Carraci (1560–1609), to describe some of his stylised portrait drawings. His example was followed by many of his immediate artistic circle and successors, but like Carraci, caricature was regarded among them as a form of amusing distraction from their main occupations as serious artists and draughtsmen.

The work of the professional caricaturist did not emerge until the early 18th century and only reached England by the 1740s, introduced initially by English amateurs influenced by visiting Italy on the Grand Tour. But during the course of the 18th century the caricature was transformed from an exclusive dilettante amusement into a powerful form of social and political critique. William Hogarth is regarded as the founder of this English tradition for his penetrating satirical portraits of types and individuals in his works on moral subjects. His skill in the treatment of the universal themes of human frailty and particularly his portrayal of well known characters, social attitudes and fashions anticipated the concerns of major artists of the late 18th century, even though he viewed with disdain aspects of contemporary caricaturists' art such as the anthropomorphic representation of human characters.

The popularity of the earliest English caricatures (or, perhaps more accurately what may be called graphic satire), was largely confined to a relatively affluent and literate audience, determined by a knowledge of the culture and attitudes of the particular world which the images depict.[1] Prints produced in the period following Hogarth were based on the works of a small number of artists. These visual satires ridiculed stereotype characters, individuals and events almost exclusively familiar to this relatively narrow social group. At the high cost of at least sixpence for black and white and two shillings for a coloured print their circulation must have been limited. Although drawn by amateurs these were usually engraved and published by the professional engraver and print seller and supplied through around half a dozen London print shops.

Towards the end of the 18th century, the fashion for caricatures was marked by the proliferation of amateur prints (particularly the mezzotint), and the broadening scope of the graphic satire to cover social and political subjects of wider significance. Works undertaken and produced by artists and publishers such as Matthew and Mary Darly, Robert Dighton and George Moutard Woodward established a taste and market for graphic satire that prepared the way for the sophisticated talents of Thomas Rowlandson and James Gillray and his successor George Cruikshank. During the Regency period, their works of social and political satire dominate what is recognised as the culmination or 'golden age' of British caricature.

By the end of the reign of George III, British satirical art had begun to lose some its pre-eminent vigour, eclipsed by French artists such as Daumier, Monnier and Philipon. In apparent reaction to its early savagery, the British caricature seemed to move towards a less vulgar and vicious form of humorous art. It was a tradition that arguably never regained the artistic accomplishment and impact of the work of Gillray and his contemporaries, in spite of the continuing popularity of the work of indigenous artists such as the Heaths and the Doyles. The publication of political and social sketches (or what came to be known as cartoons), persisted and even flourished, including the production of a significant number of medical and pharmaceutical images, notably the forceful works of C. J. Grant.

Publications such as Punch, founded in 1841 and Vanity Fair, founded in 1868, established a medium for the caricature which ensured its survival. Increasingly reproduced not as individual prints, the caricature found an outlet in satirical journals, albums and periodicals. The Victorian interest in graphic comic art has continued into the 20th century although widely challenged by new forms of mass communication satire. It has developed modern forms of expression, best illustrated by the simple and direct style of newspaper lampoon and the strip cartoon.

Images of Pharmacy and Medicine in Caricature

Caricatures which incorporate medical and pharmaceutical images form part of many major studies covering the entire field of satirical art. These range from works that explore the 17th century origins of the caricature to the many publications on 18th and 19th century British graphic satire from Hogarth onwards. In particular, the work of M. Dorothy George and the definitive catalogues of the British Museum collections provide a fairly comprehensive survey of medical and pharmaceutical subjects within the context of British social and political satires of the period.

Works from various European countries and America are covered in a number of general surveys and, more specifically, in a series of publications that concentrate on medicine and pharmacy in political prints.[2] In addition, a number of published temporary exhibition catalogues have dealt with aspects of pharmaceutical and medical iconography. Yet most of these have chosen to treat pharmacy as only part of the wider subject of medicine and cover all forms of art and illustration, including caricature or graphic satire.

Together such works cite the majority of the images of the Royal Pharmaceutical Society's collection, but for the most part based on illustrations drawn from a disparate selection of public and private sources. In general, published works have chosen to concentrate on the contribution of the caricaturists' art to our historical knowledge of pharmacy, emphasising specific details of therapeutic practice and the portrayal of the pharmaceutical practitioner and his professional role. In contrast, little consideration has been given to the pharmaceutical image within the broad tradition of graphic satire; its place within the artistic evolution of the genre or its relationship to the political and social culture of its time. With the exception of a few notable studies of individual works, the task has been hindered by a lack of detailed information available about these images. A catalogue of the Royal Pharmaceutical Society's collection cannot claim to fully remedy this situation though it should help provide evidence necessary to address these issues.

Within the scope of a collection devoted exclusively to medical and pharmaceutical caricatures, the Society's is probably only comparable in this country to the material held by the Wellcome Institute for the History of Medicine, the Victoria and Albert and the British Museums. Outside the United Kingdom, the most important permanent collections of British prints incorporating medical and pharmaceutical subjects are held by the National Library of Congress and as part of the Clement C. Fry Collection of Medical Prints and Drawings of Yale University. The Society's collection is unique, however, in concentrating entirely on the subjects of pharmacy and its association with the practice of medicine. Many of the prints are well known in the wider context of social and political satire but their inclusion here is determined by the pharmaceutical or medical interest of the particular image. By far the greatest proportion are of English origin dating from the early 18th to the mid 19th century, covering works by most of the major satirical artists of the period. The collection is based primarily on reproduced works intended to be published as individual prints, thus largely preceding the era of graphic satire reproduced in mass circulation newspapers and journals that commenced during the later 19th century. It also includes a modest selection of Continental, predominantly French prints, and a small number of original drawings. Most of these are amateur cartoons and sketches incorporated into the collection because of their special significance to the history of the Royal Pharmaceutical Society.

Origins of the Collection

In common with parts of many specialist museum collections, responsibility for the formation of the Royal Pharmaceutical Society's caricature collection belongs predominantly to one individual: Agnes Lothian Short joined the Society as Librarian in 1940 and until her retirement in 1967 devoted much of her energies to the development of the Society's collection. Her foresight and collecting activities transformed a small institutional collection of commemorative items into a substantial historical archive and museum. The rapid growth of parts of the Society's collection at this period appears to have been prompted by a small number of isolated and incidental gifts. Though for the most part these comprised modest donations and bequests of single objects, they inspired a remarkable antiquarian interest in the history of pharmacy that led to an unparalleled period of expansion and development for the Society's museum.

Under her direction the museum grew in many areas, notably in the collection of pharmaceutical ceramics and mortars. But her interpretation of the study of pharmacy extended to almost every conceivable type of pharmaceutical artefact and publication. Prior to the mid 1950s the Society had gathered only on a small scale various examples of pictorial material; a selection of commemorative and historical portraiture of distinguished pharmacists, topography and engravings after original works of pharmaceutical subjects. Primarily intended to adorn the walls of offices and meeting rooms of their former premises in Bloomsbury Square, these had been acquired as gifts, bequests, bought by subscription and occasionally purchased.

The caricature collection began in a modest way with the donation of a Gillray print, presented by the daughter of a former pharmacist in 1945. In succeeding years a number of individual gifts, including a series of prints from the L'Ordre National des Pharmaciens de France, made important additions. Only from the mid 1950s did Agnes Lothian Short commence collecting seriously in this area. During this period prints were bought at a prodigious rate; singly or in lots of anything up to 20 prints at a time, often for the more common images at a cost of only a few shillings.[3] Much of her knowledge in this area arose from the cultivation of a circle of collectors, dealers and fellow curators and this is clearly reflected in the creation of this collection. It seems evident that she recognised the financial and historical expediency of creating a collection at this time. Material was still obtainable and relatively inexpensive and thus in less than a decade the major part of the collection was acquired.

Historical Background

The medical and pharmaceutical images of this collection illustrate a period of considerable change within the professions, a process that on occasion is closely observed in contemporary social and political satires. Major steps in the demarcation of medical and allied practitioners took place in Britain, commencing towards the end of the 18th century but coming to fruition over the succeeding half century. Although the structure of the profession was eventually clarified by legal statute, licensure, formal education and qualifications, the preceding years of professional and commercial rivalry exposed the established medical world as in need of reform and regulation. This era can no longer be regarded as a period of gradual improvement and accommodation for the interests of medical traders and practitioners; instead it saw fierce conflict and competition among these groups, (including those outside the recognised medical 'estate'), arising from the struggle to establish rights and monopolies to the practice of physic and surgery and the sale and supply of medicines.

Not least among these developments was the rise in status of the dispensing druggist or chemist and druggist to that of the profession of pharmacy. The druggists, who up until the end of the 18th century largely confined their business to wholesaling, compounding and retail sales found themselves in growing competition with the apothecary. For in spite of this trade, the apothecary still held by law exclusive rights to dispense the physician's prescription. The physician in turn held authority to inspect their shops as well as exercise control over the quality of drugs they supplied. In practice only a small section of society could afford the consultation and prescription of a physician, qualified by a university medical degree and membership of the Royal College of Physicians. Instead, increasingly the apothecary met the needs of their customers who in addition to the purchase of medicines, sought as patients their services as a general medical adviser or practitioner. The conflict this created led ultimately to legislation that brought legal resolution but in the process saw an important re-alignment of interests among the traditional medical world and the gradual exclusion of those outside the orthodox and professional ranks of qualified practitioners.

Members of this established medical order were not the only form of medical practitioner operating at this period, borne out by the evidence of contemporary prints. Many emphasise the lack of distinction between the recognised physician, surgeon or apothecary and the irregular or quack. Apart from the recognised figures of the medical profession, a variety of midwives, corn cutters, nurses, herbalists and itinerant purveyors of proprietary remedies were all competing to offer their services to treat the ailing but often mistrustful public.

This era also marked the start of an important transformation in medical knowledge. Based in classical humoral pathology, the medical practice of physicians of the 18th century was rooted in a complex theoretical system which owed virtually nothing to either an empirical or a modern scientific approach to medicine. Consequently, standard diagnosis and treatment bore little relation to modern ideas of disease. Instead it would involve the application of abstract systemised concepts of disease and the use of a limited range of therapeutics, accordingly. The traditional practice of the surgeon, and the apothecary as well as the dispensing druggist might involve the observation, examination and administration of treatment while the physician could undertake his consultation without feeling the need to touch or even see their patient. However, gradual advances in scientific medicine and growing understanding of the value of clinical and pathological research date from the beginning of the 19th century. This marked the start of a rise in standards of medical practice, education and knowledge. Some of the developments that followed were met by initial public scepticism and resistance but in time led to substantial improvement in all aspects of professional health care available to the public.

Against this background, caricatures depict all ranks of the medical practitioner, ranging from the established figure of the physician to the quack or irregular. It would be misleading to imply that the image of the caricaturist is informed by a specialist knowledge of the social and professional distinctions of the medical world but as the subject of their art even the stereotype of the caricature is of significance. For these provide a source of lay observation, a visual document that reproduces not only the view of the non-specialist but one most probably taken from personal evidence and experience, that, in fact, of the sufferer and patient.[4]

In the overall context of graphic satirical art, the medical or pharmaceutical figure is most often depicted as a foil to a scene of political significance, or alternatively as part of the marginal or background interest in an image of general social comment. By contrast, only a small proportion of satires focus directly on medical issues or the practitioner, but those which do can provide an interesting popular impression of their subject. Part of their value lies in their commentary on the social rank of various medical groups, reflecting a period of transformation in public perceptions as well as attitudes to professional identity. Broadly, the content of the prints mirror these developments, not only in recording the altering status and rising aspirations of the individual practitioner but, in some images, the competition and professional rivalry that arose from these circumstances.

Central to the genre of medical and pharmaceutical images in caricature in the late 18th and early 19th century is the idea of quackery in medicine. This pervades not only the personification of the medic, but the whole concept of the medical treatment they promote and is as true for the view they depict of the diagnosis and treatments prescribed by the established physician as the irregular. Equally, those prints which focus on the actual behaviour and values reveal little respect for any type of practitioner, whether a qualified physician, a surgeon or a more lowly apothecary, druggist, mountebank or maverick itinerant. In part this is due to the apparent lack of professional and social distance established between the medical practitioner of the 18th century and the laity. Most patients would regard their own knowledge of illness and treatment as sufficient to diagnose their condition, and often prescribe and prepare an appropriate treatment. Hence, they viewed with scepticism the claims of both educated practitioners and quacks to possess either specialist knowledge or to provide 'secret' remedies. As observed through the medium of caricature, every medical or pharmaceutical type is, on occasion, seen as an object of ridicule and thus depicted as the charlatan figure or quack.

Eighteenth and early 19th century attitudes to medical men contrast with our contemporary image of the pharmacist or doctor who is rarely portrayed as the subject of a contemporary caricature or cartoon. By comparison with the comic and eccentric figures of these caricatures, doctors and pharmacists today tend to be identified as figures distinguished by their status and expertise and seem largely to escape the attention paid by cartoonists to politicians, royalty or media personalities. One explanation may be that the modern medical and allied professional is now regarded as a more credible figure, associated with specialist access to a knowledge of medical technology and pharmacy, from which, for the most part, the public are excluded. In other words today's health practitioner is seen by society as an established, virtually unimpeachable figure whose position is secured by the institutionalised bureaucracy of modern health care, one whose very respectability makes him a rare and poor subject of contemporary satire.

Ill health and the search for relief and a cure provides a rich source of metaphoric and literal imagery for the caricaturist. An illustration or an illusion to at least some aspect of the traditional treatments prescribed, sold and administered (for instance, the application of blisters and enemas, blood letting, purging, emetics, sedatives and stimulants), is recorded in virtually every medical or pharmaceutical caricature. Often this can be identified in an image by the paraphernalia of physic, particularly the apparatus of the clyster and the bottle of medicine which are employed repeatedly. But it is also portrayed in the characterisation

of the patient and the medic and in the rituals that mark their relationship, those of consultation, examination, diagnosis and the administration of medicine or a treatment.

Caricatures which satirise the claims for advances in medical science and radical new forms of treatment, such as the introduction of smallpox vaccination, betray a paradoxical sense of popular interest, incredulity and suspicion. The ineffectiveness of medical treatments, such as the cures in vogue for cholera during the 1830s, is a constant theme and one that combines scepticism for medical theory with a mockery of public naievety for their willingness to collude with these ideas. Similarly, some of the caricatures on the subject of proprietary medicines combine a satire of popular gullibility for the claims of products such as Morison's Pills and the immoral exploitation of this ignorance by their purveyors. In this instance the attack is directed not at the medical profession but, conversely, at the promotion of a product that sought to undermine the orthodoxy of conventional medical advice and treatment. Yet again we see how the comment of the caricature demonstrates a spirit of independence. From the satirical viewpoint, no area of medical practice or entrepreneurial activity

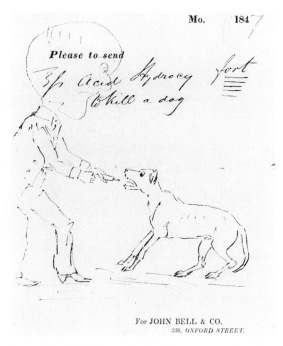

For JOHN BELL & CO.
338, OXFORD STREET.

One of Jacob Bell's comic sketches on an order of John Bell & Co.

is exempt from criticism, a situation that underlines the persistant ambivalence of the position that the caricaturist strives to achieve.

A small number of the images in this collection extend beyond the classic period of British caricature. These cover a selection of continental prints, particularly examples of the great tradition of French political caricature. In addition a distinct group of original works, including personalised sketches that appear in private correspondence or sketches that were intended for reproduction in periodicals, relate to the development of the Royal Pharmaceutical Society of Great Britain. While these fall outside the mainstream of professionally produced, popular graphic satire they depict a dimension of amateur and personal fashion for the caricature, a legacy of its origins in country house art. For instance, one notable pharmacist exponent of caricature was the founder of the Pharmaceutical Society, Jacob Bell, whose hallmark in surviving correspondence and papers is often the witty and playful sketch.[5] Thus, the development of the caricature demonstrates the complex way by which the comic rendering of familiar images is a device of both private and intimate reference as well as a powerful medium of political and social comment.

Notes and References

1. The British Museum, since the 19th century, has used the term 'satire' to describe its collections of caricature, comic art and hieroglyphical and allergorical prints. For a discussion of the distinctions in the meaning of this terminology see, for instance, the introduction to: George,

M. D., *Hogarth to Cruikshank: Social Change in Graphic Satire*, London, Viking, 1967.

2. In this context, the idea of a permanent collection refers to those held by institutions and museums rather than private individuals. Caricatures of medical and pharmaceutical interest have been widely collected and many prints cited in the catalogues of exhibited works and in the general survey anthologies on this subject belong to personal collections.

3. The level of museum documentation at this period does not provide full details of the provenance of all acquisitions though Society accounts make it clear that the bulk of the material was purchased. The great majority of prints were bought from a small group of London print dealers and antiquarian booksellers, particularly Stanley Crowe, Walter Spencer Ltd and Hugh K. Elliott.

4. The interpretation of visual images as historical records raises a variety of historiographical questions. Of these, the most important are what do the prints tell us about how the artists who produced these works viewed their subject, medicine and pharmacy, and by extension, what can the caricature tell us about the society and individuals they portray? Less easy to assess is to what extent they were intended to influence and inform rather than simply entertain? For a recent discussion of the role of the satirical print as an historical source see: Porter, R., Seeing the Past (Review Article), *Past and Present*, 1988, **118**, 186–205.

5. Jacob Bell (1810–1859), was a collector and patron of contemporary art and took an active interest in managing the business affairs of various prominent artists among his friends, including Sir Edwin Landseer RA. He held soirées for members of the artistic, theatrical and literary world and his advice was keenly sought on matters of connoisseurship and the commercial prospects of the work of many artists. It is clear that he was well acquainted with George Cruikshank. For examples of his own cartoons see annotations to *Tract No. 444*, Society of Friends Library (a bound book of religious tracts which has been annotated with a comic sketch by Bell on the fly-sheet preceding each tract) and miscellaneous letters and documents held in the collection of the Royal Pharmaceutical Society of Great Britain.

Note to Catalogue

The catalogue has been ordered chronologically by subject.

The form of each entry is as follows:

Artist and engraver if known; main title followed by transcription of subtitles and publishers', artists', and engravers' lettering, and process.

Dimensions are given in centimetres, height proceeding width.
Provenance, year and donor if known; references, descriptions and transcription of text and museum accession number.

Bibliographical abbreviations:
Standard catalogues on the works of the principal artists have been given in abbreviated form, but will be

found in full in the main bibliography.

Other abbreviations:
Prov.: Provenance
Ref.: References
WM: Watermark
[   ]: Text within square brackets is not apparent on the catalogued item and is inferred from other sources.

THE CATALOGUE

PORTRAITS OF OCCUPATIONS AND INDIVIDUALS

The traditional view of the medical practitioner depicted in caricatures is of a figure of limited expertise but low cunning with a considerable skill in persuading his patients of his powers of diagnosis (23). Though frequently depicted as a stock humorous character, this perception is not without some validity. In reality the medical practitioner for most of this period had negligible scientific medical knowledge and with only very limited choice of medication or treatment at his disposal, frequently offered little hope of providing an effective cure. Thus, it is inevitable that inflated and unrealistic claims of such figures, especially the quack or irregular, was a common and repeated source of satire (12). It has been pointed out that the satire which attacked the medical professions during the height of British caricature was less fierce than those that portray the other established professional groups, the church and the law, as well as public political figures. However, this is a view that excludes the significant number of images that employ the metaphorical use of the medical figure (for instance, the medical consultation as the parallel to the political debate or consultation), and the large number of comic caricature portraits that strictly lie outside the scope of graphic satire.

A visual impression of certain aspects of the social and professional developments that characterised this period can be traced through the prints that portray the medic or pharmacist: in particular, the transformation of the itinerant medical trader into the comparatively affluent professional figure, often marked by his translation to the position of the proprietor of his own premises (46). While many of the portraits appear to illustrate the anonymous type, a number depict specific individuals. In particular, certain notorious quacks and discredited medical practitioners who were the object of well documented and widespread public interest are recorded as the subject of contemporary caricatures.

The majority of the portrait images date from the 18th and early 19th century and it is conspicuous that there are few comparable simple portraits among the later prints. These focus on the individual figure, either a specific character (28), or a recognisable type (16). The apothecary, physician, surgeon and quack are all portrayed in comic style with their features, posture and physiognomy distorted to match the perceived character of their profession or trade, exemplified, above all, by their comic state of learned contemplation (5). Employed as a clue to identification but also to reinforce the stereotype image of their subjects, many are portrayed holding, brandishing or even administering treatment with medical instruments and preparations. The style and manner of dress and accessories, especially in the portraiture of physicians provide an additional source of satire (7). The physician who is described as having '. . . a gilt headed cane, a black suit of cloathes, a wise mysterious face, a full-bottomed flowing peruke and all other externals of his profession', *Pompey the Little* (1752, by Francis Coventry), is repeatedly mocked for his conservative attire and attitudes while the aspiring apothecary or irregular practitioner is often portrayed clumsily apeing the fashions and behaviour of his social superiors.

MAURON

1 **Mountabanck. / Le Charlatan. / Il Ciarlatano.**
65
P Tempest exc : Cum Privilegio [n.d. late 17c]
Mauron delin:

Engraving hand coloured, 25.00 × 16.70 cm.
Prov.: Purchase 1977

A portrait of the traditional travelling quack with a tame performing monkey on a rope. He stands facing holding a bottle of medicine in one hand, a medicine chest at his feet and more bottles in his pockets.

PZ. 169

ANON.

2 **Femme d'apoticaire, / eine apoteckerin,**
90
Cum. Priv. Maj. / Mart. Engelbrecht excud. Aug. V. [n.d. c. 1700]

Engraving and etching hand coloured, cut to 45.50 × 34.50 cm.
Prov.: Donation 1955, Ordre National des Pharmaciens de France

Lettered below design in French and German:
"1. un chapeau orné de fleurs. 2. boëtes. 3. boëtes. 4. verres. 5. petit mortier. 6. pilou. 7. une phiole. 8. toutes fortes de Simples. 9. une bouteille. 10. une poële. 11. un fourneau de fer. 12. une tête de mort."

This is a restrained example of a more typically seventeenth century artistic conceit, that of evoking the image of a trade in human form. Both the female apothecary and the apothecary of no. 3 are composed of items of everyday use in an apothecary's shop. The lady's torso is formed of a brass mortar, and medicine bottles and drug jars are strung around her shoulders, and medicinal plants and herbs are figured in the scene. At her feet is a skull, a reminder of death.

Companion to no. 3 (PZ. 189).

PZ. 188

ANON.

3 Un Apoticaire. / Ein Apotecker.
89
Cum. Priv. Maj. / Mart. Engelbrecht excud. A. V. [n.d. c. 1700]

Engraving and etching hand coloured, cut to 45.50 × 34.50 cm.
Prov.: Donation 1955, Ordre National des Pharmaciens de France

Lettered below design in French and German:
"1. Vase pour la Conserve de l'opiat. 2. toutes fortes de boëttes à medicines. 3. verres à medecine. 4. Lesars, viperès, serpens. 5. Patule. 6. Cirinque. 7. Cruche. 8. goblet d'or à prende medecine. 9. recepte. 10. fourneau. 11. mortier. 12. Pilon. 13. aloë. 14. Simples."

In this design, the apothecary is formed from drug jars, spatulas, a syringe, leech jars, a furnace, and glass medicine bottles. He is also set in a landscape of medicinal plants. He wears the usual leather work apron.

Companion to no. 2 (PZ. 188).

PZ. 189

ARLAUD, Jacques Antoine (1668–1743)
engraved by "S"

4 Apotekeren / l'Apothicaire
S: fc: chez C; [n.d. c. 1730]
Arlaud inv:

Engraving, 22.20 × 15.40 cm.

A young, thin and bespectacled apothecary kneels in profile to the right, his wig fallen back on his head, eyes staring, and lips pursed as he prepares to apply a hugh clyster syringe to an unseen lady – only her discarded shoe is visible next to a steaming jug. His cocked hat lies at his feet.

PZ. 143

HOGARTH, William (1697–1764)

5 *The* Company *of* Undertakers
["'CONSULTATION OF PHYSICIANS'"]
Price Six pence
Publis'd by W. Hogarth March the 3ᵈ. 1736,

Etching, 26.20 × 17.90 cm.
Ref.: Stephens, F. G., 3, i, 1877, no. 2299
George, M. D., Hogarth to Cruikshank: Social

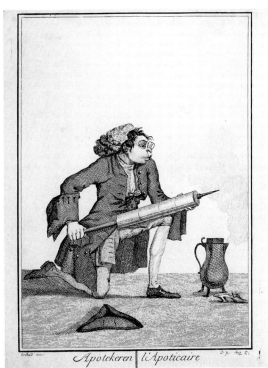

Un Apoticaire.   Ein Apotecker.

3

4

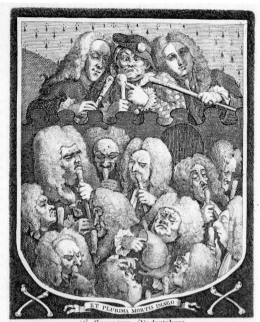

5

figures in the upper third of the shield design are portraits of three notorious quacks, on the left is the
absurd 'Chevalier' John Taylor (c. 1708–1772), the
oculist or 'Ophthalmiator, Pontificial, Imperial, and
Royal', whose cane is marked with an eye and who
leers with one eye shut at Mrs 'Crazy Sal' Mapp the
bone-setter, dressed as a Harlequin who points at her
bone-shaped staff. On the right is Dr Joshua 'Spot'
Ward (1685–1761), so-named from a facial birth
mark.

The lower part of the shield is occupied by character
studies of twelve pompous doctors, most of whom
sniff the heads of the canes in affectations of profound
thought. One holds a full glass urinal, the contents
of which he is about to test by taste, while two colleagues peer at it through their spectacles. All the
medical men wear dark suits and full-bottomed wigs.

For a later copy see also no. 31 (PZ, 82).

PZ. 81

WATTEAU, Jean-Antoine (1684–1721)
etched by POND, Arthur (d.1758)

6 Prenez des Pilules, prenez des Pilules.
Watteau del.
AP [Pond, Arthur, d. 1758] *fecit 1739*
Dr Misabin. [sic]

Etching, cut to 28.80 × 20.90 cm. Waterstained
WM : W[I?]
Prov. : Purchase

Change in Graphic Satire, London, 1967, pp.
36–7
Paulson, R., 1965, no. 144

Second state.
Lettered below design:

"ET PLURIMA MORTIS IMAGO"

"Beareth Sable, an Urinal proper, between 12 Quack-
Heads of the second & 12 Cane Heads Or, Consultant.
On a *Chief **Nebulae, Ermine, One Compleat Doctor
issuant, checkie sustaining in his Right Hand a Baton
of the Second. On his Dexter & sinister sides two
Demi-Doctors, issuant of the second, & two Cane
Heads issuant of the third; The first having One Eye
conchant, towards the Dexter Side of the Escocheon;
the Second Faced per pale proper & Gules,
Guardent,———
With this Motto—————Et Plurima Mortis Imago.

*A Chief betokeneth a Senatour or Honourable Per-
sonage, borrowed from the Greek, & is a Word signi-
fying a Head; & as the Head is the Chief part in a
Man, so the Chief in the Escocheon should be a
Reward of such only, whose High Merites have pro-
cured them Chief Place, Esteem, or Love amongst
Men. Guillim.
**The bearing of Clouds in Armes (saith Upton) doth
impart some Excellencie."

Here in this imaginary coat of arms, Hogarth satirises
physicians and quacks, and their spurious learning,
through the idiocies of Heraldry. The three half

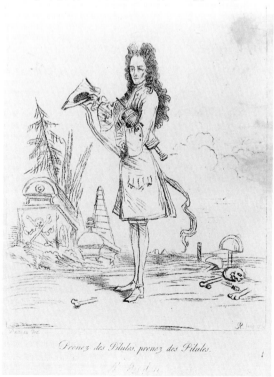

Prenez des Pilules, prenez des Pilules.

6

Ref.: Stephens, F. G., 2, 1873, no. 1987
Holländer, E., *Die Karikatur und Satire in der Medezin*, Stuttgart, 1921, p. 244

Portrait of John Misaubin M. D. (d. 1734), quack and Licentiate of the Royal College of Surgeons (admitted 25th June 1719), shown as tall and thin, facing to left, standing in a graveyard among monuments and scattered bones. Under his left arm he carries a large clyster syringe, he holds his hat in his left hand, the arm extended pointing to a monument. Misaubin was a particular target of Hogarth's graphic satire (see nos. 123 and 124), and was the subject of the satirical dedication to the play 'The Mock Doctor' by Henry Fielding (1707–1754).

The younger Angibaud, a Huguenot apothecary associated with a fine bell-metal mortar in the Museum collection, was the nephew of Madame Misaubin, the quack's widow.

PZ. 127

ANON.
etched by ?DARLY, M.

7 MON^R. LE MEDICIN.
2,
Pub^d. accord^s. to Act of Parl^l, June 13th: 1771 by MDarly 39 Strand.,

Etching and engraving hand coloured, 15.40 × 10.70 cm.
Prov.: Purchase
Ref.: Darly, M., *24 Caricatures by Several Ladies. Gentlemen Artists, &c*, Strand, London, 2, pl. 17
Stephens, F. G., 4, 1883, no. 4670

A portrait satire of the fashionable French doctor as an absurdly supercillious Macaroni, burdened with every conceivable fashionable accessory. In profile, facing left, with an exaggerated and contrived gesture he takes snuff with his left hand from a large snuff-box in his right. His coat, waistcoat and cuffs are heavily-trimmed with lace, his stockings are patterned and he wears a high crowned bag-wig. Under his left arm he carries a large parasol, which partly obscures a large fur muff, and he wears a gentleman's sword. Only one detail reveals his true profession: a clyster sticks out of his pocket with a label: "Unne Lavement pour Mademoiselle Mimi", otherwise he is the embodiment of the, "Maccaronies who trip in pumps and with Parasols over their heads". (Mrs Montague, *Her Letters and Friendships*, ed. R. Blunt, 1923, II, p. 81).

Matthew Darly issued six sets of 24 'Caricatures' between 1771–1773, which were later re-issued in six volumes, at the height of the Macaroni craze of 1770 to 1773. The word 'Macaroni' was "a term of reproach to all ranks of people who fall into absurdity" (*Macaroni and Theatrical Magazine*, October 1772). Macaronis adopted extravagant and brightly coloured, dress of elaborate hairstyles, bag-

wigs or long queues, and short, very tight frock coats and small hats (to some extent influenced by the Prussian military *neustil* then sweeping the army). Muffs carried out-doors by men were regarded as slightly foppish, and though used indoors "a decent smallish muff that you may put in your pocket" (Horace Walpole, *Correspondence*, X, Yale, pp. 144, 146) was to be preferred.

PZ. 44

[?DIGHTON, Robert (1752–1814)]

8 THE BOTANIC MACARONI
V5 11
Publishd as the Act directs Novr. 14th. 1772 by MDarly, 39 Strand.,

Etching and engraving hand coloured, 17.50 × 12.50 cm.
Prov.: Purchase 1960
Ref.: Darly, M., *24 Caricatures by Several Ladies Gentlemen Artists, &c*, London, 5, 1772, pl. 11
George, M. D., 5, 1935, no. 5046
George, M. D., *Hogarth to Cruikshank: Social Change in Graphic Satire*, London, 1967, p. 59

A finished, full length portrait of a smiling (Sir) Joseph Banks, in frock coat and breeches, wearing a bag-wig, studying a mounted plant specimen in his right hand, from which depends a briar walking stick, with a magnifying glass in his left. His right leg is swollen with gout.

Banks had only recently returned from an expedition to Iceland with Solander. This image is in marked contrast to the more usual, formal and rather severe representations of Banks.

PZ. 38

ANON.
etched by ?DARLY, M.

9 THE MACARONI . APOTHECARY,
V5 15.
Pub^d by MDarly accord^s to Act Novr 20. 1772

Etching hand coloured, 17.80 × 12.60 cm
Prov.: Purchase 1960
Ref.: Darly, M., *24 Caricatures by Several Ladies Gentlemen Artists, &c*, London, 5, 1772, pl. 15

Individual portrait, full length, of a figure with a long queue and small cocked hat, facing right adopting an exaggerated, swaggering pose, with his arms behind his back, inside his long, voluminous coat.

PZ. 147

MANSERGH R. St. G. (d. 1797)
etched by ?DARLY, M.

10 MATTHEW MANNA. A COUNTRY APOTHECARY.
Pub^d. Accor^d. to Act Octr. 11 1773 by MDarly Strand R S^t. G. Ma[nsergh] pinx^t.

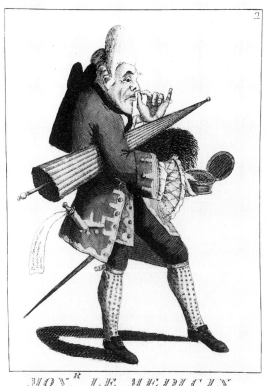

MON.^R LE MEDICIN.

7

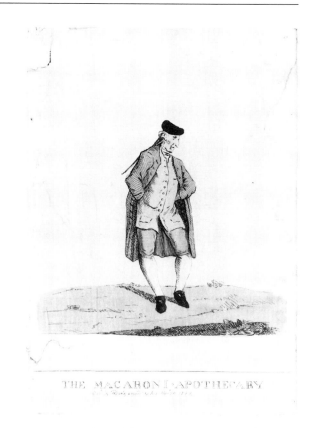

THE MACARONI APOTHECARY

9

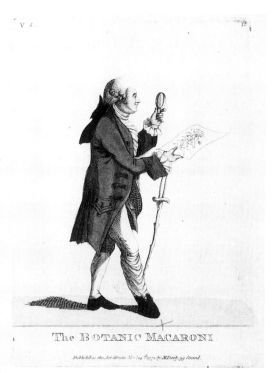

The BOTANIC MACARONI

8

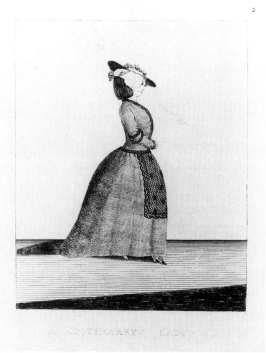

11

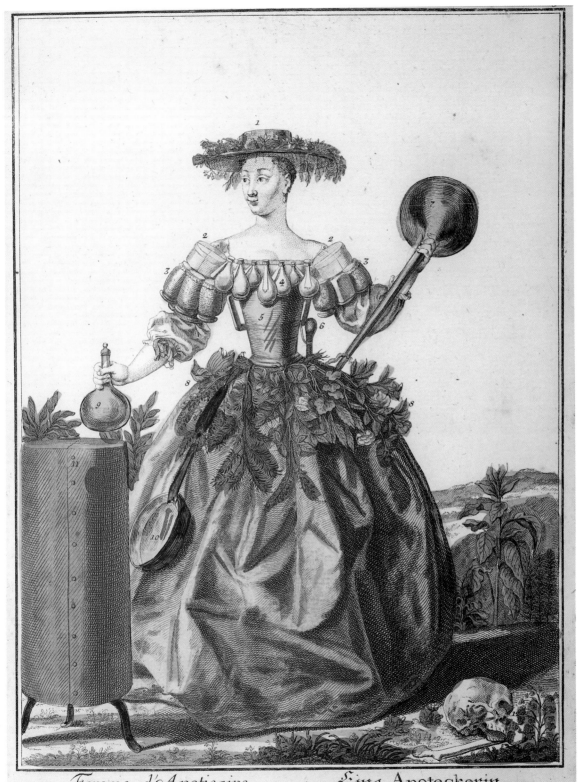

Femme d'Apoticaire.   Eine Apoteckerin.

1. un chapeau orné de fleurs. 1. ein Huth mit Kräuter geziert. 2. boëtes. 2. Schachtlen. 3.
boëtes. 3. Büchsen. 4. verres. 4. Gläser. 5. petit mortier. 5. ein kleiner Mörser. 6. pilon.
6. der Stösel. 7. une phiole. 7. eine Phiole. 8. toutes sortes de Simples 8. allerley köst-
liche Gewächse und Kräuter 9. une bouteille. 9. eine Bouteille. 10. une poêle. 10. eine Pfanne.
11. un fourneau de fer. 11. ein eiserner Ofen. 12. une tête de mort. 12. ein Todtenkopff.

Cum Priv. Maj.   Mart. Engelbrecht excud. Aug. V.

2

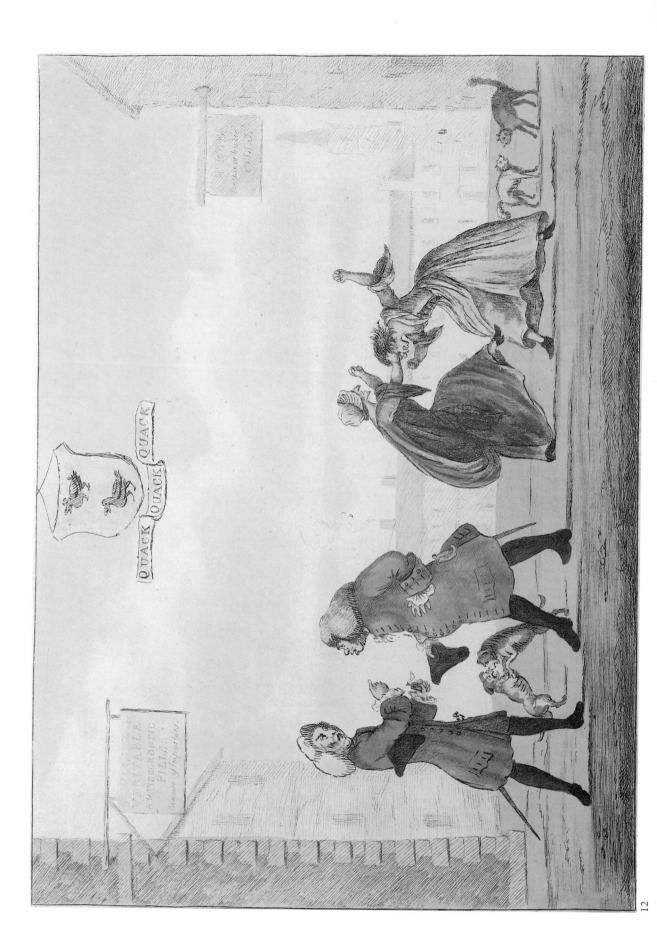

Etching, cut to 32.50 × 25.00 cm.
Prov.: Purchase
Ref.: Hein, H., Pharmacy in Caricature, Frankfurt, 1964, no. 48

In this rather naively executed satire on the humble nature of a country apothecary, the apothecary appears as an ungainly figure in a large old-unfashioned long coat with deep boot cuffs and a large, irregularly cocked hat (typical of tradesmen). He holds a wig, a staff, and has a ?barber's bowl under his arm. His shop is depicted as a rough, single-storey thatched, stone cottage. For illiterate customers, as was common practice, it has a sign, a prominent barber's pole (see also no. 124), while a board above the single window proclaims:

"MATT MANNA Apothecary, surgeon, CORN Cutter &c &c, Man midfife [sic], Gentlemen shaved & Hogs Gelded, shave for a penny & Bleed for 2 pence".

Through the window can be seen outlines of an anatomical skeleton, a wig stand, and a man being shaved. Outside the window are two dishes and a drug jar labelled "JALAP".

PZ. 94

ANON.
etched by ?DARLY, M.

11 An APOTHECARYS LADY
V3 2.
Pub^d. by MDarly 39, strand Jany. 1. 1774

Etching, 25.30 × 17.70 cm.
WM: VI
Prov.: Purchase 1960
Ref.: Darly, M., 24 Caricatures by Several Ladies Gentlemen Artists, &c, London, 3, 1774, pl. 2

Portrait satire on the pretensions of the Apothecary's wife, shown in profile walking to right, hands clasped at waist, dressed in the height of fashionable 'undress'. Her face concealed by large straw hat (tilted forward over eyes by her hairstyle), the latest style of round cap beneath, and wearing a gauze or embroidered apron. On same proof sheet as no. 13 (PZ. 154. 1).

PZ. 154

BUNBURY, Henry William (1750–1811)
etched by BRETHERTON, James (fl. 1770–1790)

12 MUTUAL ACCUSATION.
Publish'd by Bretherton &^rd. January 1774.
Mr Bunbury del.
J^s Bretherton f

Etching hand coloured, cut to 38.50 × 43.70 cm.
Ref.: George, M. D., 5, 1935, no. 5279

Lettered below design:

"When once you've told & cant recall a lye
Boldly, percist in't or your fame will die

Learn this ye Wives, with unrelenting Claws
Or right or wrong, Assert your husbands cause".

Above design, below a shield decorated with two ducks the motto:

"QUACK QUACK QUACK"

A street scene showing two warring households, the rival quacks, the wives, and their dogs and cats each fight one another in the road between their two competing premises, the shop sign on left lettered:

"DR WALKERS VERITABLE / AИTISCORBUTIC / PILLS. / Beware of Impostors".

Shop sign on right: "TRUE antiscorbutic PILLS".

The arguing quacks, one thin the other stout, are shown in frock coats, carrying cocked hats, with 'physical' wigs and armed with dress swords. The image of the fatter quack is very similar to no. 15 (PZ. 153). Their wives, however, attired in common-wear gowns, are actually fighting, kicking, and pulling one another's hair.

PZ. 5

ANON.
etched by ?DARLY, M.

13 A Meek-aroni Hornpipe —
V. 3 6,
Pub according to Act by Mdarly 39 Strand May 24th 1774

Etching, 25.10 × 17.70 cm.
WM: VI
Prov.: Purchase 1960
Ref.: Stephens, F. G., 4, 1883, no. 4708
Darly, M., 24 Caricatures by Several Ladies Gentlemen Artists, &c, London, 3, 1774, pl. 6

Portrait of stout man facing, doing an energetic dance, holding his cocked hat in his left hand, a cane in his right. He wears a tight frock coat, and tie-wig. On same sheet as no. 11 (PZ. 154).

PZ. 154. 1

WIGSTEAD, Henry (d. 1793)
etched by Rowlandson, Thomas (1756–1827)

14 THE VILLAGE DOCTOR.
[Pubd H Humphrey Bond St 1774]
Etching and aquatint cut to 25.00 × 19.50 cm.
Prov.: Purchase 1958
Ref.: George, M. D., 5, 1935, no. 5274
George, M. D., Hogarth to Cruikshank: Social Change in Graphic Satire, London, 1967, pp. 95–97

At a house with a sign of a pestle and mortar above the door and a board proclaiming "PROBE SURGEO[N AND] MAN MIDWIFE". The village doctor, in nightshirt and cap, his breeches in his left hand, leans out of a upper window angrily shaking his right fist at the anxious and hatless man standing below who has woken him.

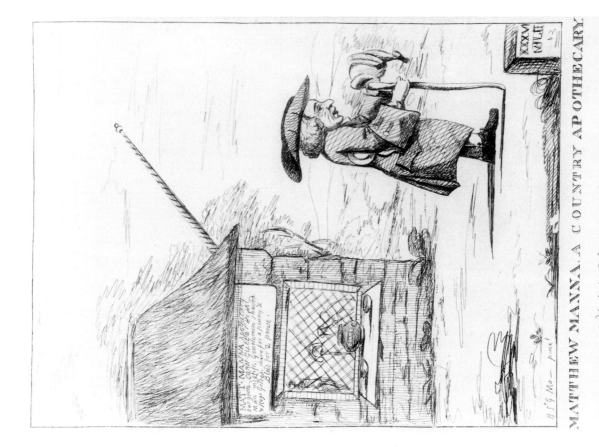

The subject was suggested by Henry Wigstead and his initials are depicted on a fence to the right of the door.

Artist's and publisher's names have been partially trimmed away.

PZ. 109

ANON.
etched by ?DARLY, M.

15 The bruising Apothecary – paratus operi — ,
V3 2
pub by MDarly 39 strand Sep . 1 . 1774

Etching hand coloured, cut to 21.00 × 16.00 cm.
Prov.: Purchase
Ref.: Darly, M., 24 Caricatures by Several Ladies Gentlemen Artists, &c, London, 3, 1774, pl. 2

One of the later issues of Darly's series of ''Macaroni'' prints. A portrait of a coarse, stout man standing pugnaciously in profile facing to the right. His left hand is clenched into a fist, his shaved head is bare since he has torn off his large 'physical' wig (almost a universal symbol of the medical man), which he holds in his right hand, to be ready for the fray. He wears a very large greatcoat and clumsy shoes with large fashionable buckles. The colouring is not original.

For a similar treatment of the irascible apothecary see also no. 12 (PZ. 5).

PZ. 153

LOUTHERBOURG, Phillippe Jacques de (1740–1812)

16 From Warwick Lane,
London, Printed for R. Sayer & J. Bennet N°. 53 Fleet Street, as the Act directs 26 Dec'. 1776.,
P.I. de Loutherbourg Fecit
Torre Excu'.

Etching, 16.00 × 11.70 cm.
Prov.: Purchase 1960
Ref.: George, M. D., 5, 1935, no. 5361

A re-issue by Sayer of a satirical portrait produced by Torre. It shows a bizarre figure in profile facing to left, said to be a caricature of ''a well known M.D., one of the last remaining of the old school'' (George, op. cit.). He is shown as a very thin man wearing an excessively tight yet very old-fashioned full-skirted frock coat and a huge wig that conceals much of his cocked hat and face – around which buzz five flies. His neck is covered by a high stock, his chin is unshaven. He carries a silver-topped cane in his right hand, his left in his pocket and wears a dress sword.

See also no. 19 (PZ. 90), for a later issue.

PZ. 89

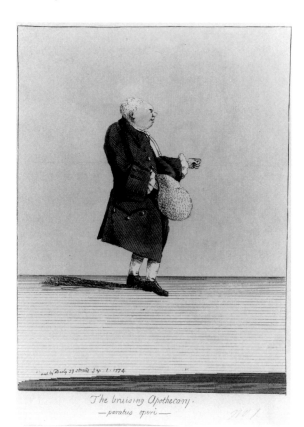

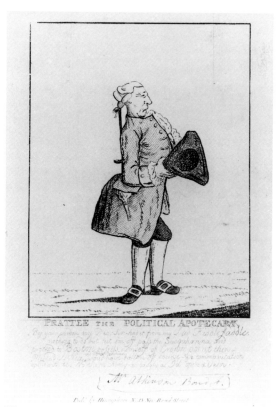

15

17

[?] GILLRAY, James (1756–1815)

17 PRATTLE THE POLITICAL APOTECARY,
Pub^d. by HHumphrey N°. 18 New Bond Street [n.d. c. 1779]
Signed in ink: Mr Atkinson Bond St. [sic]

Etching, 24.90 × 17.70 cm.
Prov.: Purchase
Ref.: George, M.D., 5, 1935, no. 5603A

Lettered below design:

"Beg your pardon my Dear Sir – had it from my Lud Fiddlefaddle, nothing to do but cut 'em off pass the Susquhanna and proceed to Boston possess himself of Crown point then –Philidelphia ^and South Carolina, would have fallen of course – & a communication opend with the Northern Army – as easyly as I'd open a Vein''.

Portrait of a thin, elderly and haughty man wearing a full-tailed frock coat, with a bag-clyster in one pocket. William Atkinson, an apothecary whose premises were on Pall Mall, gives a considered, and no doubt valuable, opinion on the British strategy for the later stages of the American War of Independence.

A different version was published by Darly on 12th August 1779.

PZ. 83

[?] GILLRAY, James (1756–1815)

18 APOTHECARIES_____TAYLORS, &c Conquering FRANCE and SPAIN.
[Publisher illegible: W Humphrey 227 Strand] [n.d. c. 1779]
[J. Gillray ?]

Etching hand coloured, 26.00 × 36.30 cm.
WM: J WHATMAN (PZ. 70)
Ref.: George, M. D., 5, 1935, no. 5614

A large group of tradesmen, including a barber (who wears a comb in his wig, and has a powder-puff in his pocket), a shabby tailor (with scissors in his pocket) and the apothecary William Atkinson, sit and stand at a round table in a tavern room, drinking punch and giving their opinions of the current political situation – the possible French and Spanish invasion.

The image of Atkinson is no. 17 (PZ. 83), reversed.

The ingratiating Prattle says to the barber:

"Beg your Pardon my Dr Sir meant no Offence my Dr. Mr Tallow – too much Love & Respect – your Perfectly in the Right – of the same Opinion of my [––]ed &c J[–––] they'll never Invade us as you say &c my Lod Chatter [–––] to me the other Night at my Lady Carbuncl[es]''

Colouring differs between the two copies.

PZ. 70
PZ. 71

LOUTHERBOURG, Phillippe Jacques de (1740–1812)

19 From Warwick Lane,
London, Pub^d, by Willm. Holland N° 50, Oxford Street May 1st. 1790,
P. I. de Loutherbourg Fecit
Torre Excut.

Etching hand coloured, cut to 14.40 × 10.30 cm.
Prov.: Purchase 1960
Ref.: George, M. D., 5, 1935, no. 5361

A later re-issue of no. 16 (PZ. 89) by Holland.

PZ. 90

NEWTON, Richard (1777–1798)

20 AN APPARITION.
London Pub^d. W. Holland N°. 50 Oxford Street May 1 1790.
Newton del

Etching and aquatint hand coloured, cut to 49.50 × 37.50 cm.
Prov.: Purchase 1959

A tall, grim and ghostly figure in shroud and tall cap stands by a grave in a night churchyard. A grave-robber, with round brimmed hat, pick and spade at his feet by a skull and bones, holds up a lantern in horror.

PZ. 132

NEWTON, Richard (1777–1798)

21 RESURRECTION MEN,
London Pub Octr 1 1792 by W Holland N°. 50 Oxford Street
[D]esigned& Etch'd by R Newton
Newton del

Etching and aquatint hand coloured, cut to 51.00 × 37.80 cm.
Prov.: Purchase 1958

A night scene, three grave-robbers, with hair standing on end in terror, in the act of raising a coffin are surprised by a ghostly shrouded spectre. One man is kneeling hauling on the rope, one holds a lantern, one stands and directs the work.

PZ. 97

ANON.

22 D^r. VE–––D–––N,
WONDERFUL MAGAZINE.
Gratis___ to the purchasers of the Wonderful Magazine_____Pub^d. by C. Johnson. [c. 1793]

Engraving, 17.00 × (cut to) 12.20 cm.
Ref.: Wonderful Magazine, i, 1793, p. 406
      George, M. D., 7, 1942, no. 8371

Second state copy of an earlier issue.

This portrait satire is of Miss "Chevalier" John

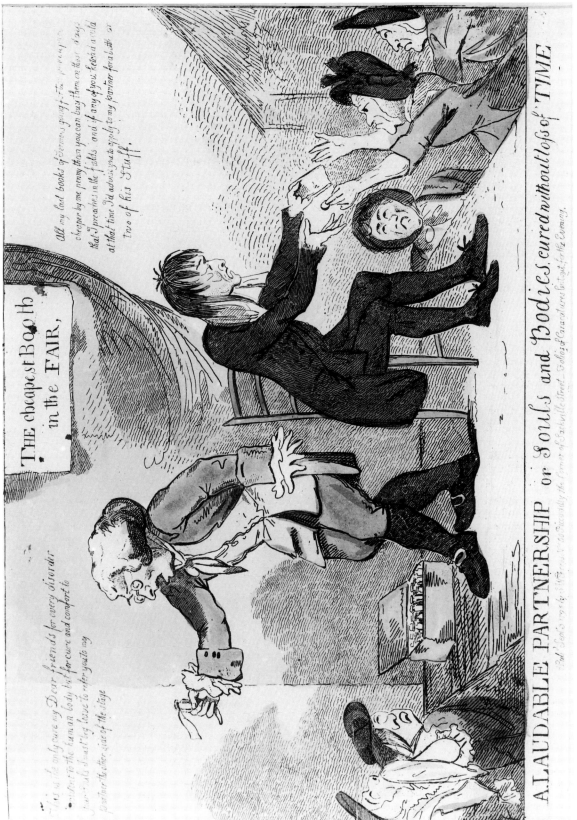

Theodora de Verdien, a noted London eccentric and transvestite. Similar portraits were published after her death, on 16 July 1802.

An elderly 'man' in a large coat, wearing bag-wig and cocked hat, walks stooping, in profile to the left towards the entrance of a bookshop, two large books under the left arm, an umbrella under the right, a walking stick in his right hand and pockets filled with books. Prints and notices are displayed in the shop's window: "Old Books Bought", and "Price 6[—] Import[ant] Life of Paine".

Lettered below scene:

"A remarkable Walking Bookseller Quack Doctor &c. &c.
hawking Old Books as Mosess do Old Cloaths.
Stop Gentle Reader, & Behold
A Beau in Boots, searching for Gold,
A Walking Bookseller, an Epicure,
A Teacher, Doctor & a Connoisseur".

A pamplet "*Important Memoirs of the life of Thomas Paine*" was published in 1795.

William Holland had a Print and Caricature Warehouse at 50 Oxford Street between 1782–1803, and was imprisoned for one year and fined £100 for selling Paines '*Letter to the Addresses*' in 1793.

PZ. 142

ANON.

23 A German Quack Doctor,
[n.d.]

Etching and ?aquatint hand coloured, cut to 28.10 × 17.00 cm.
Prov.: Purchase 1960
Ref.: Holländer, E., Die Karikatur und Satire in der Medezin, Stuttgart, 1921, p. 257
Weber, A., Caricature Médicale, Paris, 1936, p. 73

Lettered below design:

"Here my good Friends is de grand Specific for all de disorders incident to de Human body."

A smiling foppish doctor, in profile facing right, wearing a frock coat and a bag-wig, leans forward ingratiatingly indicating the labelled bottle of medicine in his left hand.

PZ. 155

[?WOODWARD, George Moutard (1760–1809)]

24 A LAUDABLE PARTNERSHIP or Souls & Bodies cured without loss of TIME
Pub^d Septr 3 1795 by S W Fores N° 50 Piccadilly the Corner of Sackville Street—Folios of Caracatures lent out for the Evening.

Etching hand coloured, cut to 22.00 × 34.00 cm.
WM: E & B
Prov.: Purchase 1958

Ref.: George, M. D., 7, 1942, no. 8741

Below a sign "THE cheapest BOOTH in the FAIR", a quack and a dissenting preacher address an audience of five country women from a stage. The quack, wearing spectacles and a 'physical' stands facing left and holds out a bottle of medicine, saying:

"This is the only cure my Dear friends for every disorder incident to the human body but for cure and comfort to your Souls I must beg leave to refer you to my partner the other side of the stage"

His companion the preacher, his hair disordered, wearing bands and dressed in grey, sits on a chair facing right and passes a paper to a customer in exchange for a coin:

"All my last books of Sermons going for two pence a piece cheaper by one penny than you can buy them on those days that I preaches in the fields and if any of you ketch'd a cold at that time I'd advise you to apply to my partner for a bottle or two of his Stuff."

PZ. 130

WOODWARD, George Moutard (1760–1809)

25 Fleabottomi
[S W Fores 50 Piccadilly] [n.d. c.1798]

Etching hand coloured, cut to 20.00 × 14.70 cm.
Prov.: Purchase 1960
Ref.: Genuine Orthography Candidates for public favour, May 29 1798

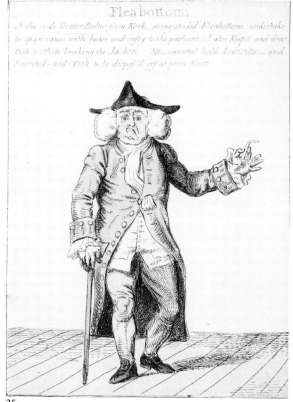

25

Full length portrait of a man, his face with a particularly vacant expression, standing facing. His left arm outstretched holding out a lancet, while resting on cane in right hand. He wears a long coat fastened by one button, his long cravat tied in a very old-fashioned 'steinkirk' (the end passed through a button hole), and an unkempt powdered wig under a cocked hat. He declares:

"I the reale Doctor Bolus from Kork, aving studid Fleabottomi, undertaks to opan vanes with hease and safty to the pashunt, I also Kups, and dras Tith withote braking the Ja bon. NB___savaral hold Lancitts___and Saccond-and-Tith, to be disposs'd off at prim Kost,."

PZ 131

WEST, T.

26 AN ADDRESS of THANKS from the Faculty to Right Honble, Mr INFLUENZY for his kind visit to this country.
Pub^d, April 20th, 1803 by S W Fores 50 Piccadilly _____Folios of Caracatures lent out
T. West del^t,

Etching hand coloured, cut to 22.50 × 33.50 cm.
Prov.: Purchase
Ref.: Holländer, E., Die Karikatur und Satire in der Medezin, Stuttgart, 1921, pl. 2
Zigrosser, C., Medicine and the Artist, New York, 1970, no. 93

This satire attacks the excessive profit perceived to be made by doctors out of suffering, and their corrupt practices. A group of nine doctors, one with spectacles, one a Scot, all dressed in sombre 'professional' grey, argue as to the efficacy of their rival remedies, and bow and kneel as they come before the personification of Influenza to present their "ADRESS OF THANKS", they say:

"I humbly hope when our worthy Friend takes his departure, he will leave some few of his relics behind, for our future Benefit."

"My Friend Mr Newbery made me a very handsome present for my recomendation of his James's powders in the Newspapers" (Newbery was the sole agent for James's powders, see no. 95, 'The Magazine's Blown Up').

The Scotsman has a letter in pocket, lettered: "accoacheur to the most exalted rank at Weymouth & elsewhere", and says: "Hoot Mon, we have naw ha[d] sic a Friend many a gud Day."

"D---r . . . I hate . . . Glaubers . . . Ginger I say"

"Twas the opiates did the good"

"Should be happy to set you down in my new chariot Mr influenzy"

"My prescription of angelica root & nitre"

"It was Broadburns, Syrup of Butterflies was superior to everything."

Influenza is depicted as a thin, elderly man in a nightcap, a shade over his eyes, and a nightshirt, seated on a commode. A bandage is pinned around his neck. On a table beside him are bottles labelled "Opening Draught", "Sweating Draught", "Emetic", a large flagon of "Laudanum", a sealed package of "James's Powders", and a clyster. Below the table is a barrel of "PERUVIAN BARK", and a large carboy of "GARGLE".

PZ. 128

WOODWARD, George Moutard (1760–1809) etched by CRUIKSHANK, George (1792–1878)

27 The SAILOR and the QUACK DOCTOR!!
Pubd. by T. Tegg 111 Cheapside, [n.d. c. 1807]
Woodward del
Cruikshank Sp

Etching hand coloured, 24.50 × 34.80 cm.
Prov.: Purchase
Ref.: George, M. D., 8, 1947, no. 10896

A satire against quacks and their improbable claims of cures. A sailor in typical land rig of striped trousers, short jacket, neckchief and wide-brimmed hat is shown in consultation with a quack in his room. Behind him in a cabinet hangs an anatomical skeleton. Under his right arm the sailor carries a wooden club (he is possibly with the press), in this hand he holds a "List of Cures", his left eye is bandaged. He says, in a satire on nautical jargon:

"You must know Doctor I have got a bit of a Confusion on my larboard cheek from a chance shot, and as I dont think it of consequence enough for our Ships surgeon, I bore down to you, after overhauling a long list of your cures – but I suppose from the messmate in the Cabin there, you dont always make a return of the Killed and wounded."

With his left hand in his pocket and pointing with his right to a pen and paper on a table, the quack, dressed in frock coat, breeches, embroidered waistcoat and powdered wig, replies:

"Sir, my rule of practice is this, there is pen, ink, and paper, – sign a certificate of your cure, and I'll take you in hand immediatly on paying down two Guineas!"

PZ. 126

DIGHTON, Richard (1795–1880)

28 IRELAND in SCOTLAND or a trip from OXFORD to the land of Cakes.
Drawn Etch'd & Pub^d. by Dighton, Char^s Cross, J[une 1807]
[Date of publication erased]
Signed in ink: Mr Ireland

Etching hand coloured, 27.10 × 19.60 cm.
WM: [–] E---] (PZ. 39); 1814 (PZ. 40)

Ref.: George, M. D., 8, 1947, no. 10783

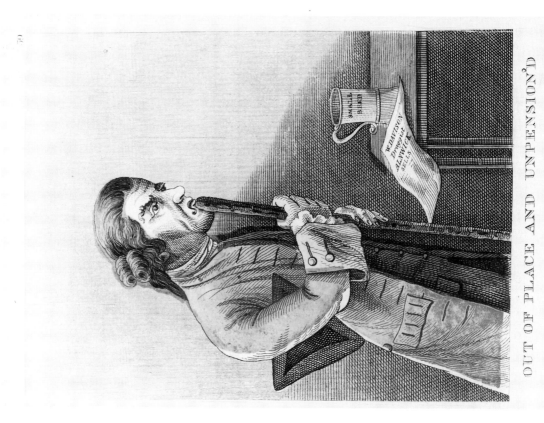

OUT OF PLACE AND UNPENSION'D

Printed and Published by W. Davison-Alnwick.

32

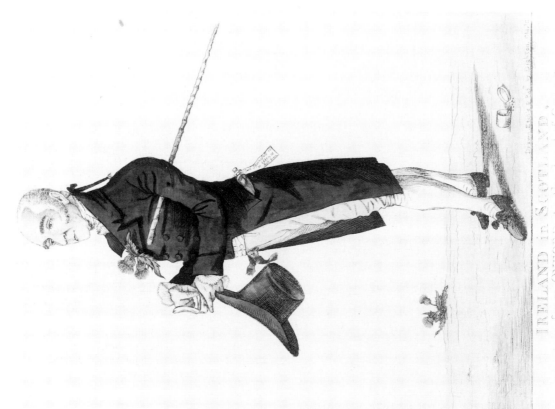

IRELAND in SCOTLAND,
... trip from OXFORD to the land of C....s.

28

Portrait of John Ireland M.D., depicted as a fashionable man standing directed to the left. He wears a large thistle in his buttonhole and carries a cane under his arm. A medicine bottle in his pocket has a label lettered: "Two spoonfull to be taken at bedtime."

Dighton was invited to Oxford by a Dr Grosvenor, Taunton, and Hall specifically to produce this caricature of Ireland.

Colouring of the two copies differs slightly.

PZ. 39
PZ. 40

WOODWARD, George Moutard (1760–1809)
etched by "CW"

29 THE CHEERFUL COBLER
by Thos, Tegg 111 Cheapside, [n.d.]
Woodward delt.
CW Sculpt
Price one Shills Color'd

Etching hand coloured, 24.80 × 35.00 cm.
WM: W[HATMAN] TURKEY MILL
Prov.: Purchase

The scene is a village street, on the far side of the road is a half-timbered house with a signboard of a pestle and mortar and two coats of arms, lettered: "JOHN HEAVEN Apothecary and UNDERTAKER". Next to this is a thatched cottage with a sign above the door: "Abraham Amen Parish Clerk and Sexton", and the owner in the doorway.

In the foreground a cobbler sits working on a bench outside his shop and recites a nonsense rhyme: "When a twister a twisting will twist him a twist . .", while two sailors in shore rig listen, one says: "Scuttle my Hammock Jib if this here fellow does not beat our Parson.", and the other replies: "I think so Messmate and the Surgeon into the bargain." In their opinion all three talk meaningless nonsense.

PZ. 129

ROWLANDSON, Thomas (1756–1827)

30 DOCTOR GALLIPOT placing his Fortune at the feet of his Mistress, Thro' Physic to the Dogs
Published by Reeve & Jones No. 7, Vere Street Novr 1, 1808
Rowlandson

Etching and aquatint hand coloured, cut to 43.00 × 36.50 cm.
Prov.: Purchase 1956
Ref.: George, M. D., 8, 1947, no. 11114

One of a set of copies of watercolours by Rowlandson. An unattractive, foppish apothecary with 'grog-blossemed' profile kneels at the feet of an attractive young woman, one hand on his breast, the other pointing to a cloth at his feet on which are spread syringe and bag clysters, spatula knife, pestle and mortar, and a large bottle: "Elixir of Life DROPS". She stands in some confusion and alarm, while behind an open door a highly amused man observes the scene. In the background are the curtains of a bed.

PZ. 100

HOGARTH, William (1697–1764)
engraved and etched by COOK, Thomas (1744–1818)

31 CONSULTATION OF PHYSICIANS
ET PLURIMAMORTIS IMAGO
Published by Longman, Hurst, Rees, Orme, Jany. 1st, 1809.
Hogarth pinxit.
T. Cook sculpt.

Engraving and etching, 27.70 × 22.50 cm.
Ref.: Newton, J., and Stevens, G., The Genuine Works of William Hogarth, London, 1810, ii, facing p. 144

A later copy, reversed, of no. 5 (PZ. 81).

PZ. 82

ANON.

32 OUT OF PLACE AND UNPENSION'D
39
Printed and Published by W. Davison, Alnwick. [n.d. c. 1810]

Engraving uncoloured, (PZ. 37) and coloured, by stencil (PZ. 36) 23.30 × 17.00 cm. (PZ. 36, trimmed to platemark).
Prov.: Purchase

Three-quarter length portrait of a preoccupied man, in an old-fashioned frock coat, his hair tied in a queue, a cocked hat under his right arm, facing to right leaning thoughtfully on a long staff, before him a table bearing a flysheet headed: "W. DAVISON Druggist ALNWICK SELLS", and a mug lettered: "SMALL BEER".

The enterprising William Davison (1781–1858), published some 42 caricatures in the style of Darly and Gillray during the first few decades of the nineteenth century. A chemist and druggist in Alnwick from 1802 Davison had after 1808, following a partnership with the printer John Catnach, become in addition a noted stationer, printer and publisher.

Interestingly, one of the impressions has been coloured by means of a poorly registered stencil, which suggests that Davison might have had difficulty in securing the necessary skilled colourists in Alnwick.

PZ. 36
PZ. 37

ROWLANDSON, Thomas (1756–1827)

33 MEDICAL DISPATCH OR DOCTOR DOUBLEDOSE KILLING TWO BIRDS WITH ONE STONE

TEGG'S CARICATURES Nº 47
Price One Shilling Coloured
Rowlandson Del

Etching hand coloured, cut to 50.50 × 39.50 cm.
Prov.: Purchase 1956
Ref.: George, M. D., 8, 1947, no. 11638
  Holländer, E., Die Karikatur und Satire in der Medezin, Stuttgart, 1921, p. 241
  Weber, A., Caricature Médicale, Paris, 1936, p. 91

An old, invalid woman sits senseless in an arm-chair directed to the left. A doctor, stout and middle-aged, with a cane "MEDICAL STAFF", takes her pulse, while putting his arm round a plump young woman who leans on the back of the chair. They gaze eagerly into each others' eyes. On a table is a bowl of "COMPOSING DRAUGHT", and a pillbox "OPIUM".

PZ. 105

ROWLANDSON, Thomas (1756–1827)

34 THE LAST GASP OR TOADSTOOLS MISTAKEN FOR MUSHROOMS

Pubd. September 1st, 1813 by Thos Tegg Nº 111 Cheapside
Price One Shilling Coloured

Etching hand coloured, cut to 33.00 × 23.00 cm.

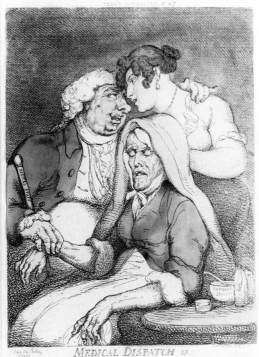

MEDICAL DISPATCH OR
DOCTOR DOUBLEDOSE KILLING TWO BIRDS WITH ONE STONE

33

Prov.: Purchase 1956
Ref.: George, M. D., 9, 1949, no. 12145

An elderly old-fashioned doctor with gold-topped cane and spectacles sits bending forward and peers myopically at the tongue of a fat agonized patient sitting in a low armchair to the right beside his thin and ugly wife. A scrawny footman, hair standing on end, stands behind the doctor's chair, the heads grouped against a high window. A longcase clock on the left shows the time is 2.22. A thermometer hangs on the wall opposite.

PZ. 103

ANON.

35 [Untitled]

A Paris chez Jean, Rue St. Jean de Beauvais Nº. 10.
[n.d. c. 1800–20?]
Signed with Dutch translations of the French captions:
chimist in zyn laboratorium, kunstenaar, wand-heeler, horlogiemaker, kleevhourrer, slachter.

Engraving hand coloured, 20.50 × 28.40 cm.

Six illustrations depicting the practice of an unusual selection of occupations, entitled: "Chimiste dans son laboratoire", "Phisicien", "Chirugien"," horloger", "Boucher", and "Chaircuttier". The surgeon is placed above the butcher in the series. The "Chirugien" is shown as a young, well-dressed man letting blood into two bowls set on a small table from the forearm of an attractive and fashionable young woman in cap and gown, who reclines on a couch in front of a screened bed.

PZ. 141

DIGHTON, Richard (1795–1880)

36 THE MARKET MENDS

Drawn Etchd. and Pubd. by Richard Dighton June 1822
Signed: Mr Mends Druggist

Etching hand coloured, cut to 23.50 × 17.00 cm.
Prov.: Purchase
Ref.: George, M. D., 10, 1952, no. 14415

Full length portrait in profile of a prosperous druggist, Mr Mends standing to the right wearing a top-hat, and dressed in a long single-breasted brown coat over white trousers. A wall forms the background.

PZ.35

MONNIER, Henri (1805–1877)
Lithographed by DELPECH, Francois-Seraphin (1778–1825)

37 Apothicaire,

Hi Monnier [1824]
[–], *lith de Delpech*

Lithograph coloured, cut to 25.00 × 34.00 cm.
Prov.: Purchase

Ref.: Hein, H., Pharmacy in Caricature, Frankfurt, 1964, no. 9

An excellent depiction of the interior of a busy apothecary's of the early nineteenth century. An assistant copies out a recipe, another works in the corner near a female assistant (the apothecary's wife?), three gentlemen pass the time by the counter in front of a showcase of drug jars, a dog lies curled-up and asleep. An iron mortar on a stand is a prominent feature.

PZ. 91

LISLE, Joe

38 CHEAP MUSIC.
Pub^d. 1830, by, S, Gans, Southampton Street,.
Drawn by Joe Lisle.

Etching and aquatint hand coloured, cut to 31.80 × 21.00 cm.
Prov.: Purchase

A customer, an emaciated figure in top-hat with umbrella in a music shop, says to the fat man behind the counter, surrounded by shelves of sheet music:

"Mr. Catgut I want to purchase a Cheap Fiddle." He replies:

"Then you had better go to the next Chemist and purchase four Penny-worth of Daffy's Elixir and he'll give you a VIAL IN."

Daffy's Elixir was a famous and well-established proprietary medicine, the pun concerns the supply of the distinctive container with the product.

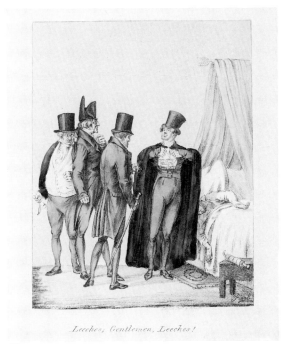

Leeches; Gentlemen, Leeches!

Text slightly blurred.

PZ. 88

PIGAL, Edme Jean (1798–1872)

39 Leeches; Gentlemen, Leeches!
London Pub^d by A Sharpe [n.d. c. 1830]
Pigal

Engraving in crayon-manner coloured, 31.00 × 23.60 cm.

On the left the patient slumps half-out of his bed, partly concealed by a doctor facing a group of three of his fellows, all but one dressed in grey, with top hats (though one is old-fashioned and wears his hair in a queue under a bicorne hat). He tears up the prescriptions of his fellows inscribed: "Good W[–––], An Emetic, Bleed him." while declaiming the title. On a small bedside table is a clyster syringe.

PZ. 106

SEYMOUR, Robert "SHORTSHANKS" (1799/1800–1836)

40 CHOLERAPHOBY.
[T MClean, 26 Haymarket] [1832]
[Seymour, R.]

Lithograph coloured, 12.00 × cut to 10.20 cm.
Prov.: Purchase 1960
Ref.: The Looking Glass, 24, 1831, London, p. 2
George, M. D., 11, 1954, no. 16931

Distraught customers crowd around an apothecary's counter. A fat man pounds with a pestle in a mortar; a fashionable shopman serves, another, with a wink, takes a drug jar from a shelf. A boy holds out a coin and says: "I wants a pennorth O camphor", an anxious woman in a large bonnet: "I feel very poorly", another cries for "Spirits of Wine and mustard", others ask for "Camphor" and call "Soap Sir".

This outbreak of cholera had first appeared at Sunderland in 1831, possibly from Hamburg, and had spread to London by February 1832.

PZ. 13

DOYLE, John "HB" (1797–1868)
Lithographed by DUCOTES, A.

41 Administering a bitter dose to a fractious patient.
HB Sketches N°. 244
Published by Thos. McLean 26 Haymarket Feb 26th. 1833
HB
A Ducotes Lithog^y. 10 St Martins Lane.

Lithograph, 20.30 × 35.40 cm.

John Bull is dosed by Peel, Grey & Castlereagh in the guise of a doctor, his assistant and a nurse. He struggles as one, tipping back John Bull's chair says: "His agitation is quite alarming. – I can scarcely keep him down." The second, measuring a dose from a medicine bottle into a spoon, declares: "These inflamatory

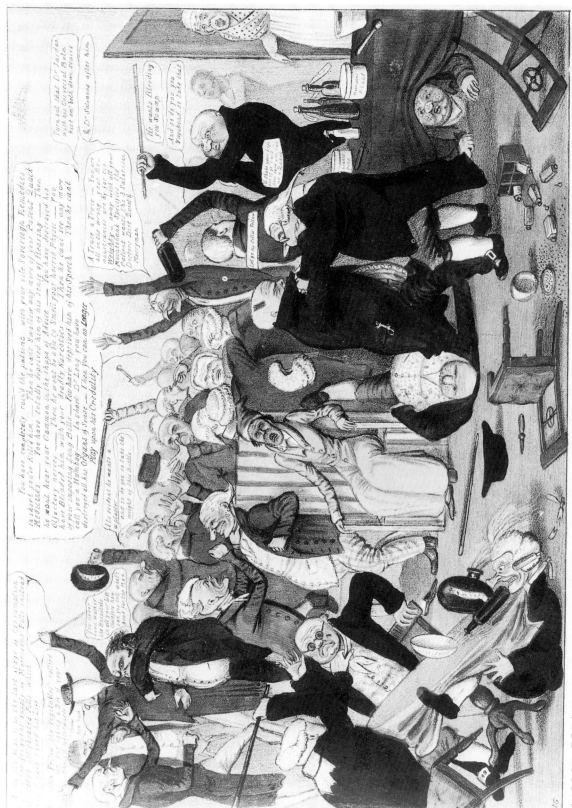

symptoms must be abated by a little counter irritation.", while the third (dressed as an old nurse with pestle and mortar), says: "See there! such a nice bit of sugar!"

Two onlookers remark: "I protest that with the exception of a slight tinge of Grey, it is nothing more than poor C−stle−gh's black draught." And: "Oh! These people will take the bread out of our mouths."

PZ. 3

GRANT, Charles Jameson (fl. 1828–1846)

42 FRONTISPIECE TO THE "DOCTOR", THE LANCET: MEDICAL GAZETTE, GAZETTE OF HEALTH; &C
London Pubd by J Kendrick 54 Leicester Squr. July 25 1833
C J Grant Invent Del & Lith

Lithograph cut to 28.60 × 19.50 cm.

A series of 25 humorous vignettes, comprising a series of rather dreadful visual and verbal puns, titled: "A Burning Inflammation", "A Galloping Consumption", "The Dropsy", "The Scarlet Fever", "The Cramp", "The Gripes", "Miss carrying", "The Small Pox", "Shortness of Memory!!", "The Scurvy!", "The Hooping Cough!".

The central scene is titled "The Stomach Complaint!", and is a satire on the general view of the efficacy of medicines. A seated druggist, writhing with legs drawn up, and grasping his stomach in agony, his face wryly contorted with pain, and saying to a surprised, bespectacled, and very old-fashioned doctor:

"Oh Doctor Doctor give me aid!
My Brain's on fire, my bowls ache
In making up some Patient's Pills
I took a couple by Mistake!!"

PZ. 76

GRANT, Charles Jameson (fl. 1828–1846)

43 SUDDEN BREAKING UP OF A CONSULTATION. Weighty Arguments on both sides! _____ When Doctors disagree, Who shall Decide.
[n.d. c. 1835]
CJG

Lithograph coloured, cut to 19.00 × 26.00 cm.

An invalid, beyond all cares, sits wearing nightgown and cap, surrounded by a great rioting mob of doctors who argue for their rival medicines, and brawl armed with their canes and even glass carboys, watched by an astounded housekeeper. Pills and bottles are scattered on the floor; on a table is a mortar and pestle and boxes of "Morrisons Pills" and "Leakes Pills", two famous proprietary medicines. The doctors are captioned:

"You have completely ruin'd the patient with your vile Sovereign Remedies in short you've Kill'd him.

_____Then he can't Swallow any more of your Patent Quack Medicines.__You have totally deprived him of his sense of Hearing.__Then he won't hear your Gammon in the shape of Advice__You have destroyed his Olfactory nerves. __Then he won't be able to Smell your horrid Physic__you have Blinded him with your deadly Narcotics__Then he can't see any more of your imposing Long Bills__You have deprived him of his Speech__Then he can't call you a Humbug−−In short Dr Long you have destroyed all his Organs of Sense__Then you can no Longer Play upon his Credulity."

"Turn out that Dr Jardan with his Universal Balm kick em' both down stairs"
"& Dr Solomons after him"

"A Truce a Truce__You are all in the wrong. Your Remonstrances are by far too Weighty__away with all your Mountebank Specifics, the patient wants the 3 Salernian Doctors, Diet, Quiet & Merryman"

"He wants Bleeding you Scamp"
"And so do you, you Vagabond. so take that"

"Let go my Collar Fellow"
"I'll shake your Life out of ye I will__how dare you call me a Quack"

"I say the man is in the last stage of Consumption thro' a too frequent supply of Morrisons Pills instead of Leakes sillybrated Pills which would have saved his Life"
"It's false Fellow, the 'Vegetables' rallied him, but taking a Box of your Rubbish afterwards threw him back"

"You never even Walked the Hospitals in all of your Life therefore how can you tell what's good for the man"

"Its evident he wants a plaster"
"And so do you so take the weight of this Bottle"

PZ. 75

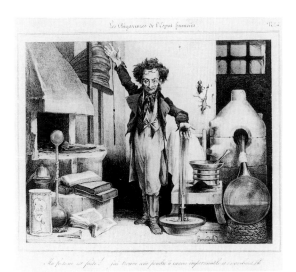

BOURDEL, Jean Baptiste Desire
lithographed by LEMERCIER

44 Les Bigarrures de l'Esprit humain N°. 4,
[Hautecoeur Martinet, Rue du Coq, Paris] [c. 1838]
Bourdel
Lithograph coloured, 19.50 × 21.50 cm.
Prov.: Purchase

Lettered below design:

"Ma fortune est faite! j'ai trouve une poudre à canon
impermeable et incombustible."

In a laboratory surrounded by alembics and chemical
apparatus the chemist, standing facing, announces
his amazing discovery of waterproof and incombustible gunpowder, the properties of which he demonstrates by pouring a quantity onto a candle set in
a basin of water. A satire on the contemporary search
for a stable form of gunpowder.

PZ. 4

HEATH, Henry (fl. 1824–1850)

45 A MEDICAL CONSULTATION
No. 33
Published by I. B. Brookes 9 New Bond St. *Sole*
Publisher of Mr. Henry Heaths Sketches [n.d. c. 1835]
H. Heath.
Printed by Lefevre & Kohler 52 Newman Street

Lithograph coloured, 22.00 × 15.70 cm.

A print satirising colloquial speech. A footman
lounges at a druggist's counter, on which there are
three large bottles. Behind the counter the aproned
assistant is at work pounding a mortar.

"Are you going to Hepsom Sam?"

"Yes if I can get an Orse."

PZ. 84

ANON.

46 NOTIONS OF THE AGREEABLE No 21.
[L]ondon W Spooner 377 Strand. [n.d. c. 1830–40]

Lithograph coloured, cut to 18.00 × 13.00 cm.

An apprentice wearing an apron over his livery
stands pounding a large iron mortar on a wooden
block and addresses the fashionable druggist who
stands behind the counter pouring from a shop round
into a medicine bottle.

"Please Sir I dont think Mister Foozle takes his Fissick
regler"

"No! Why?"____"Cos he's getting vell so precious
fast"

On the counter are bottles, a drawer from the drug
run, shop rounds and a marble mortar, the walls are
lined with drug runs and shelves for shop rounds and
drug jars. The scene is a careful depiction of work
in a contemporary pharmacy or apothecary's shop.

PZ. 172

GRANDVILLE, Jean-Ignac (1803–1847)
lithographed by BARA, J.

47 Le Pharmacien
JJ Grandville [1841]
J Bara

Lithograph coloured, cut to 39.00 × 31.00 cm.
Prov.: Purchase 1977

Full length portrait facing of the pharmacist standing
in front of a balance on a counter. He wears a long
coat and spectacles, his left hand in his pocket.

PZ. 78

GRANDVILLE, Jean-Ignac (1803–1847)
lithographed by STYPULKOWSKI

48 L'eleve de pharmacie.
JJ Grandville [1841]
Stypulkowski

Lithograph coloured, 25.00 × 18.50 cm.
Purchase

Portrait of a young assistant in an apron; he stands
behind a counter unenthusiastically pounding a
mortar. On the counter is a drug jar "SODIUM" and
a dropper. In the background is a drug run with a
drawer labelled "POTASSIUM".

PZ. 72

ANON.

49 [Oh Doctor, Doctor!]
London: Marks & Sons
[n.d. c. 1850?]

Woodcut hand coloured, 24.00 × 17.00 cm.

Lettered below design:

"Oh Doctor, Doctor! come this way:
And do not for a moment stay,
Make haste to kill both young and old,
And fill thy purse with ill got Gold,
Hark! don't you hear the Night Bell ring,
You wicked Butcher looking thing,
Pound the Pills, mix the draught betime,
You shall not be my Valentine."

A crudely executed portrait satire of a medical man
holding a huge medicine bottle in both hands, labelled "CHLOROFORM". He has a clyster in his pocket,
behind him is a large mortar and pestle decorated
with a skull motif, and three large pills lettered:
"TWO AT NIGHT", "AND ONE IN", "THE
MORNING".

Shopfittings in the background, and a shelf with
three pillboxes and two square bottles.

PZ. 162

ANON.

50 [Untitled]
[n.d. c. 1850?]

Woodcut hand coloured, cut to 24.00 × 17.00 cm.

Lettered below design:

"You man-killing poisoning creature
Here is pictured each ugly feature
Of your impudent conceited face
Which a monkey even would disgrace

Your Jalap or Rhubarb won't suit me,
And as I don't like Senna Tea,
I really, Sir, must quite decline,
To have you for my Valentine!"

A sharp-featured ugly apothecary or druggist, pounding a large mortar decorated with a skull and crossed bones, by bottles and jars of "PILLS". Waterstaining on margins.

PZ. 163

NAU, Jean

51 UN CLIENT SÉRIEUX
COLLECTION HUMOURISTIQUE 72 (on reverse)
A NOYER PARIS [n.d.]

Photomechanical coloured, 14.00 × 9.00 cm.
Postcard. Lettered below scene:

" – C'est bien ici la **Pharmacie Foirus**, ancien intenrne des Hopitaux de Paris, chimiste expert de la **Ville de Paris**, lauréat du Concours de 89, diplomé de l'Université de Chicago?"

" – Parfaitement, Monsieur"

" – Alors, donnez-moi deux sous de boules de gomme"

A short, fat and bespectacled man with an umbrella, lifts his bowler hat to a tall, thin, bearded and similarly bespectacled pharmacist (behind a counter surrounded by drug jars), and orders some pastilles after a few discreet enquiries.

PZ. 98

DISEASES AND THEIR TREATMENT

The study of the caricature provides an insight into popular perceptions of disease and its treatment from a variety of viewpoints. These universal themes appear in virtually every medical or pharmaceutical caricature but this section concentrates on those in which the main image is focused on the patients experience of illness and the effects of treatment or on the relationship between the medical practitioner and his patient.

Ill health and the role of the practitioner in diagnosing, administering or prescribing treatment is explored through a number of the most powerful of the caricatures of the collection (53). This relationship is charged with literal and metaphorical meaning that is a rich source of comic comment. Submitting to the expertise of the doctor is viewed with anything from simple humour to considerable distrust. In many of these prints the patient is seen as the helpless victim of the physician or quack and in others as his cuckold.

One of the most characteristic images of the collection is that of the personification of illness (70, 71). Various artists produced prints in which the central figure is depicted suffering from the effects of a medical condition (59, 60, 61, 87). The blue devil is a familiar device in a number of these prints (notably those of George Cruikshank), where the patient's condition is highlighted by these imaginary figures who torment him (54, 77). The blue devil is a metaphor (as well as a pun) for the malaise that he is haunted by, a character suggesting a physical, mental and psychosomatic explanation for his condition. In some images these are the very cause of their pain as it is the demon who quite literally inflicts suffering upon the patient.

The effects of medication are an equally important subject of satire. 'Taking Physic' (56, 85, 93), an image repeated in the work of a number of artists, expresses through the anguish and facial distortion of the patient the horrible taste of the medicine. This was a very real problem as many forms of oral medicine were highly unpalatable and little was effective to disguise the taste. To the patient, as depicted through the eyes of the caricaturist, the cure in the form of prescribed medication was often considered worse than the condition it was intended to treat (87, 90).

Among the selection of medical instrumentation that appears in the caricature, the eneema or clyster is one of the most frequently used images (66). This apparatus appeared to exercise considerable prurient fascination and provide a source of endless ridicule, even though it was commonly used to perform a variety of medical functions. As well as purging a variety of instruments in the form of pumps and syringes were used for administering nourishment and medication to treat a host of internal conditions.

In France its use was particularly popular and appears repeatedly in Daumier lithographs and many French prints as well as works by Gillray and other English artists. The general use of unpleasant procedures and medication were not the only source of satirical comment: Specific therapeutic developments in the treatment of disease, such as the introduction and effects of smallpox innoculation, are also the subject of some of the most pertinent caricatures of medical significance.

Images that examine the role of the apothecary and later the chemist and druggist or pharmacist serving and advising his patient, provide some of the most detailed contemporary records that survive of the context in which he worked (86). Though they often deliberately exaggerate the humour of the typical shop interior, these images still offer a valuable impression of the typical trappings of the apothercaries' or pharmacists' trade.

ANON.

52 DOCTOR BLOWBLADDER discovering the PER-PETUAL MOTION.
[n.d.]

Mezzotint and etching hand coloured, cut to 13.50 × 11.00 cm.
Ref.: Holländer, E., Die Karikatur und Satire in der Medezin, Stuttgart, 1921, pl. 7
Weber, A., Caricature Médicale, Paris, 1936, p. 92

An elderly, stout and old-fashioned doctor feels the pulse of a fashionably-dressed, demure young lady seated at his left and glances thoughtfully at her, and distractedly sniffs his cane. In his pocket is a bottle labelled: ''Blessed Medicine''.

Gum arabic has been employed in the colouring to add depth to the shadows.

PZ. 159

DUNTHORNE J.
etched   by   ROWLANDSON,   Thomas
(1756–1827)

53 AGUE & FEVER,
Pub 29th March 1788 by T. Rowlandson, No 50 Poland Street as The Act directs
Designed by James Dunthorne
Etch'd by T Rowlandson

Etching   and   aquatint   hand   coloured, 41.50 × 55.80 cm.
Prov.: Purchase 1958
Ref.: George, M. D., 6, 1938, no. 7448
Holländer, E., Die Karikatur und Satire in der Medezin, Stuttgart, 1921, pl. 6

Weber, A., Caricature Médicale, Paris, 1936, p. 70
Zigrosser, C., Medicine and the Artist, New York, 1970, no. 85

Lettered below design:

'' 'And feel by turns the bitter change of fierce extremes, extremes by change more fierce', Milton''.

Patient, teeth chattering, sits in profile to left in a well-furnished room, before a fireplace and holding his hands to a blazing fire. Ague, a sinuous, snaky monster, clings to him, while Fever, a furry monster, stalks the room.

On the right the doctor sits in profile writing a prescription and holding up a medicine bottle.

A companion to 'The Hypochondriac' published by Rowlandson in 1798.

PZ. 178

NEWTON, Richard (1777–1798)

54 THE BLUE DEVILS!,
[L]ondon Pubd. by W. Holland, Oxford Street Feb. 10, 1795.
Designed & Ethd by Rd Newton

Etching and aquatint hand coloured, cut to 34.80 × 24.80 cm.
Prov.: Purchase
Ref.: George, M. D., 7, 1942, no. 8745

An invalid, in profile to left, wearing a nightshirt sits in an armchair in front of his curtained bed. He draws away in abject terror from the sight of seven small and completely naked demons (save one who wears large thigh boots), who dance around him hand in hand in a circle. On a round table to the right are a medicine bottle and a book: ''Essay on the Power of Imagination''.

PZ. 96

GILLRAY, James (1756–1815)

55 PUNCH cures the GOUT, the COLIC and the 'TISICK.
Pubd. July 13th. 1799. by H. Humphrey, 27, St James's Street

Etching hand coloured, cut to 25.75 × 34.25 cm.
Prov.: Purchase 1957
Ref.: George, M. D., 7, 1942, no. 9449

In this piece illustrating a simple form of self-medication a trio of invalids sit around a large punch bowl on a small round table, each holds up a full glass to make a toast. A fat, gouty man in a nightgown speaks the first part of the title, a lady holding her stomach speaks the second, and a very thin man says the last.

The traditional rhyme concludes, 'And is by all agreed the very best of physic'.

PZ. 63

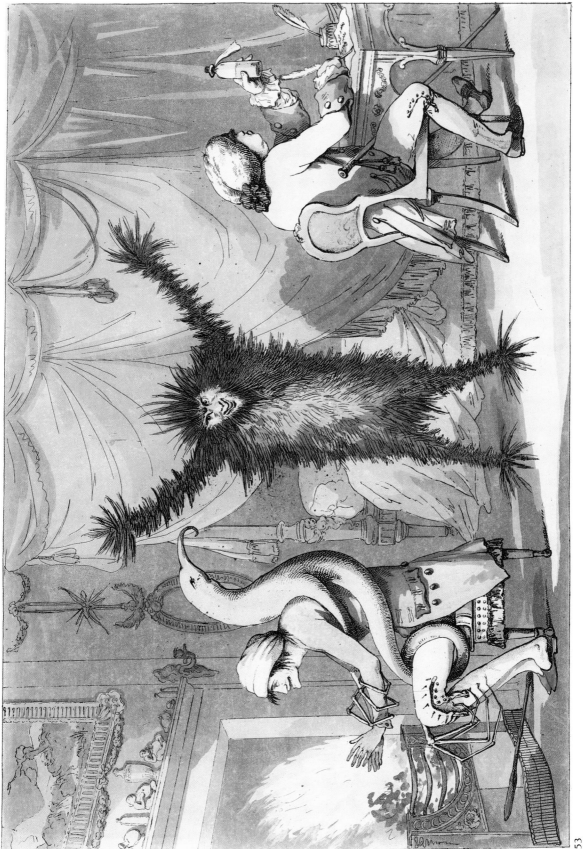

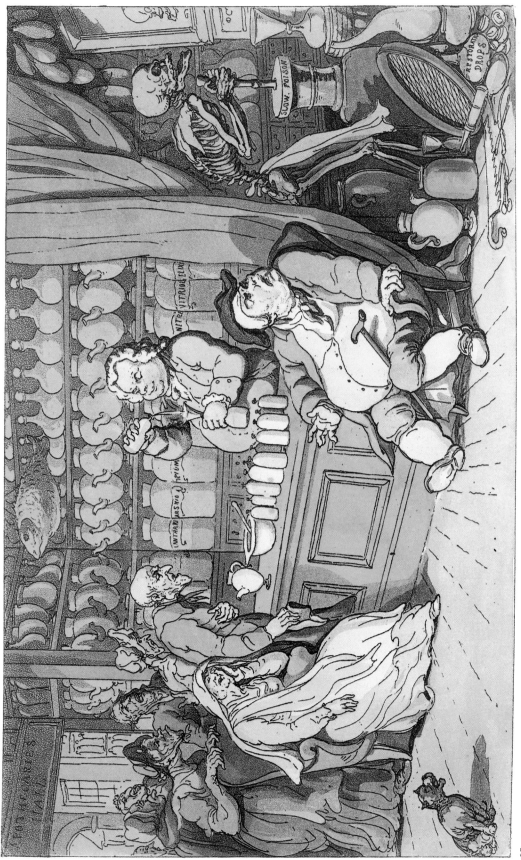

GILLRAY, James (1756–1815)

56 Taking PHYSIC.

[*Publish'd Feby. 6th. by H. Humphrey. 27. St James's Street. London.*]

Etching hand coloured, cut to silhouette 21.50 × 16.50 cm.
Ref.: George, M. D., 7, 1942, no. 9584
    Hein, H., Pharmacy in Caricature, Frankfurt, 1964, p. 24, fig. 7, 181

One of the best known, much imitated, and justly popular satires on a medical theme, a study in facial expression, which became part of a series comprising in addition nos. 60–63, and all illustrated in the window of Humphrey's print shop in no. 137 'Very Slippy Weather'.

A dishevelled, unshaven man, wearing only a night-cap, shirt, disordered breeches, and slippers, stands by an empty fireplace, his face expressing an extreme of revulsion for the taste of his medicine, he holds a medicine bottle in one hand, a full cup of medicine in the other. More medicine bottles are on the mantelpiece.

PZ. 50

GILLRAY, James (1756–1815)

57 COMFORT to the CORNS.

Pub^d. Feby. 6th. 1800. H. Humphrey 27 S^t. James's Street J^s. Gillray inv^t. & fec^t.

Etching hand coloured, cut to 23.50 × 17.90 cm.
WM: ED MEADS & CO 1809
Prov.: Purchase
Ref.: George, M. D., 7, 1942, no. 9585
    Holländer, E., Die Karikatur und Satire in der Medezin, Stuttgart, 1921, pl. 5

An old woman in a shawl sits in a carved gothick chair by a large open fireplace, sticks burn on the hearth. She leans forward, her mouth open in eager anticipation as she prepares to use a large knife to cut at her corns. Both the large string of onions on the wall, and the carved decorations on the chair resemble the corns on the woman's feet. Beside her chair are a tub, towel and scrubbing brush and by the fire is a large cat.

PZ. 55

GILLRAY, James (1756–1815)
etched by BROCAS, W

58 COMFORT to the CORNS

Pub^d. by I. Sidebotham 24 Lower Sackville S^t., Dublin [n.d.]
Etch'd by W. Brocas Junr.

Etching hand coloured, cut to 27.50 × 20.20 cm.
Prov.: Purchase 1956

A very close and competent copy of no. 57 (PZ. 55), not reversed, save the tub is shown as empty of water.

PZ. 54

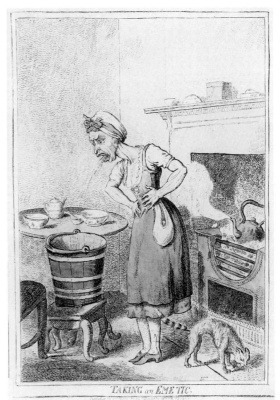

TAKING an EMETIC.

59

CRUIKSHANK, Isaac (1756–1811)

59 TAKING an EMETIC.

Published by S W Fores No 50 Piccadilly March 12 1800 IC^k

Etching hand coloured, cut to 26.40 × 18.30 cm.
Prov.: Purchase 1958
Ref.: George, M. D., 8, 1947, no. 9805

A companion to 'Taking Physic', no. 56; in the corner of a kitchen in front of a fireplace an elderly woman stands spewing into a bucket set on a stool. She wears cap, stays, and petticoat. A kettle boils furiously on the fire to her right and vomits forth clouds of steam, her cat arches and mewles as it retches. Teacups and bowls in Oriental-style are arranged on the mantelpiece and on a small round table.

PZ. 20

SNEYD, Rev. John (1766–1835)
etched by GILLRAY, James (1756–1815)

60 Brisk – CATHARTIC.

Published Jany. 28th. 1804 by H. Humphrey, St James's Street, London.

Etching hand coloured, cut to 24.00 × 18.30 cm.
Prov.: Purchase 1956
Ref.: George, M. D., 8, 1947, no. 10305

The invalid, seated facing on a water-closet, wearing his greatcoat and cap, and holding his stomach with a look of anxious and horrified expectancy on his face. A pair of breeches and stockings are on a clothes-horse in the foreground.

From the series including no. 56, and 61–63.

PZ.66

SNEYD, Rev. John (1766–1835)
etched by GILLRAY, James (1756–1815)

61 Gentle Emetic,
Publish'd. Jany 28th. 1804. by H. Humphrey. S^t. James's Street.

Etching hand coloured, cut to 35.00 × 27.50 cm.
Prov.: Purchase 1955
Ref.: George, M. D., 8, 1947, no. 10304

The invalid's head is held above a bowl on a table by a country apothecary in his riding clothes and boots with spurs. The long-suffering patient wears a nightcap and unbuttoned waistcoat.

From the series also including no. 56, and 60, 62–63.

PZ. 51

SNEYD, Rev. John (1766–1835)
etched by GILLRAY, James (1756–1815)

62 Breathing a vein,
Publish'd. Jany. 28th. 1804 by H. Humphrey. S^t. James's Street.

Etching hand coloured, cut to 35.20 × 28.00 cm.
Prov.: Purchase 1955
Ref.: George, M. D., 8, 1947, no. 10306

The operator is the same rustic apothecary, or vet, shown in no. 61 (PZ. 51) in spurred top boots. The patient sits, eyes closed.

From the series also including no. 56, and 60–61, and 63.

PZ. 52

SNEYD, Rev. John (1766–1835)
etched by GILLRAY, James (1756–1815)

63 Charming – well again,
Publish'd. Jany. 28th. 1804 by H. Humphrey. S^t. James's Street.

Etching hand coloured, cut to 35.00 × 27.50 cm.
Prov.: Purchase 1955
Ref.: George, M. D., 8, 1947, no. 10307

After his many ordeals, the recovered patient sits happily behind a table laid with a cooked fowl and eggs, he holds up a glass of wine, and both he and his liveried footman have broad smiles of satisfaction at the happy conclusion.

From the series also including no. 56, and 60–62.

PZ. 58

ROWLANDSON, Thomas (1756–1827)

64 The Last drop

Pub^d. April 5 1806 By T. Rowlandson N^r James S^t. Adelphi

Etching hand coloured, cut to 41.00 × 31.50 cm.
Prov.: Purchase 1956
Ref.: George, M. D., 8, 1947, no. 9786

An adaption of an earlier Darly issue of 1773, the figures reversed and altered. A short and fat man stands in profile to the right on tip-toe by a side table, raising a punch bowl to his lips oblivious to the bowl's supporter, death personified as a jubilant skeleton, who stands behind his victim about to plunge a spear into his head.

On the table are a foaming tankard of ale, lemons, a decanter of port, by it on the floor a row of casks, empty bottles, a corkscrew, and a flagon of "Usque baugh", the water of life.

PZ. 104

ROWLANDSON, Thomas (1756–1827)

65 The CONSULTATION or last hope
*Pub^d. May 12th 1808—by R. Ackermann N° 101 Strand,
Rowlandson inv 1808*

Etching hand coloured, cut to 42.50 × 51.00 cm.
Prov.: Purchase 1972

Lettered below design:
"So when the Doctors shake their heads, and bid their Patient think of Heaven—Alls over, good Night".

Four doctors, in old-fashioned campaign and bag wigs, one with spectacles, crowd around a gouty and bemused John Bull, who sits with each foot on a pillow. One doctor takes his pulse and listens to a watch. Two more doctors rest from their labours, seated in the background on the right, waited on by their patient's harrassed liveried servant, one carries a cane and sword, the other is in sober grey. Two parsons wait in background for their turn, a female servant stands on the left before a curtained bed.

Papers on floor: "Prescription to be shaken before taken", and: "Timothy Screwdon Undertaker Funerals Performed".

PZ. 107

ELMES William 'XYZ' (fl. early 19c)

66 JACK, hove down – with a Grog Blossom Fever.
*Pub^d. Augt 12. 1811 bt Thos. Tegg N° 111. – Cheapside – Opposite Bow Church – London,
By XYZ*

Etching hand coloured, 24.50 × 34.50 cm.
Prov.: Purchase
Ref.: George, M. D., 9, 1949, no. 11825

A thin, elderly doctor crouches by a cannon, before a brawny but invalid, inebriate and pock-marked seaman lying sick in his hammock. Both are typical caricatures in both their peculiarities of dress and in

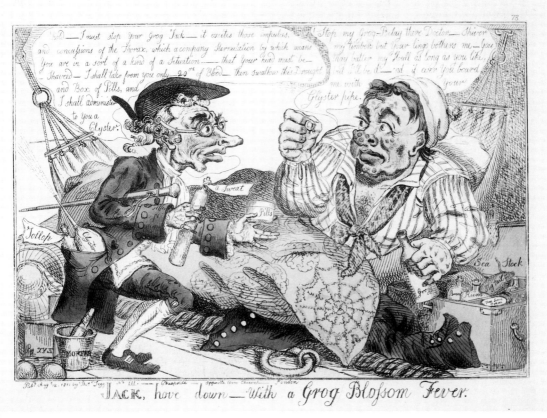

JACK, hove down—With a Grog Blofsom Fever.

66

their incomprehensible (to a layman), speech and give an interesting insight into the lay perception of both: the doctor is old fashioned in a long frock coat, wearing a powdered wig, spectacles and a cocked hat. In his left hand he carries a box of pills, in his right hand is a bottle labelled "a Sweat", a gold-headed cane is under his arm. His pocket bulges with a gushing clyster and a bottle labelled "Jollop" [sic], beside him is a pestle and mortar and two cannonballs (which at this time were commonly called "pills", for obvious reasons). He says:

" 'hold – I must stop your Grog Jack – it excites those impulses, and concussions of the Thorax, which a company [sic] sternutation by which means you are in a sort of a kind of a Situation – that your head must be Shaved – I shall take from you only – 20 ozs of Blood – then swallow this Draught and Box of Pills, and I shall administer to you a Clyster' ".

The sailor, wearing a seafarer's striped shirt and neckchief replies:

" 'Stop my Grog. – Belay there Doctor – Shiver my timbers but your lingo bothers me – You May batter my Hull as long as you like, but I'll be d____'nd if ever you board me with your Glyster pipe' ".

He shakes his large right fist at the doctor, his left holds a bottle of "Grogg", while beside him his "Sea Stock" chest contains bottles of "Rum", "Brand[y]",

a "True Love Token", and a ball of "Pig tail".

PZ. 144

ANON.
etched by "W-E"

67 SCOTCH Training for a Milling Match
Price One Shilling Coloured
16 Octr 1811. Pub^d. by Thos. Tegg No 111 Cheapside London.
W-E. Sculpt

Etching hand coloured, cut to 21.60 × 32.00 cm.
Prov.: Purchase

A young man in short jacket, a boxer in training, squats over a bucket with his breeches down; on the wall behind him hang a pair of huge hand-like gloves. He says:

"Oh"__my Guts__Captn. dont you think I am reduced enough".

A Scotsman, the boxer's trainer, wearing a bonnet with a large thistle, kneels by a large open fireplace applying a bellows to a fire under a steaming cauldron marked: 'Crowdy', replies:

"Hoot awa' man, another muckle mess of Crowdy, and a fiew Doses of Scotch Pills, will do your business".

Around him are heaped sacks and chests of "Haggis", "Oatmeal", "Bannocks", "Kale", "Scotch Barley", "Sheeps heads", "Scotch broth" and "Gruel". By the fireplace, near a recess containing a jar of "Scotch Sniff", sits a woman spinning, on the mantelpiece are containers of "Whisky", "Scotch Pills", "Flour of Brimstone" and "Treacle", and hanging from a nail is a broken "Scotch Fiddle".

The 'Scotch Pills' are probably the well-known Anderson's Scots Pills, a cathartic, produced from c. 1635 until the early twentieth century, containing aloes, anise, jalap, myrrh and gamboge.

PZ. 99

NEWTON, Richard (1777–1798)
etched by ROWLANDSON, Thomas
(1756–1827)

68 A GOING! A GOING!!!,
[date erased ?1813]
Thos. Tegg No 111 Cheapside.
R Newton del
Rowlandson f..

Etching hand coloured, cut to 23.00 × 32.30 cm.
Prov.: Purchase
Ref.: Hein, H., Pharmacy in Caricature, Frankfurt, 1964, no. 40

A fat doctor wearing old fashioned dress, a gold-headed cane under his left arm, his cocked hat under the other, stands in profile with a complacent smile regarding his dying patient seated in an armchair to the right. An old nurse stands in a doorway behind the doctor. By the patient is a small round table with a medicine bottle, a bowl and spoon and a paper lettered: "PRESCRIPTIONS BOLUS &c BLISTERS". Medicine bottles and pots line the windowsill.

The doctor declares:

"My Dear Sir you look this Morning the Picture of health, I have no doubt at my next visit I shall find you intirely cured of all your earthly infirmitys".

PZ. 95

ROWLANDSON, Thomas (1756–1827)

69 [The Quack Doctor]
London Pub. July 1–1814 at R. Ackermann's, 101 Strand.

Etching and aquatint hand coloured, cut to 33.00 × 40.00 cm.
Prov.: Purchase
Ref.: Combe, The English Dance of Death, 1, 1814, p. 85
George, M. D., 9, 1949, no. 12421

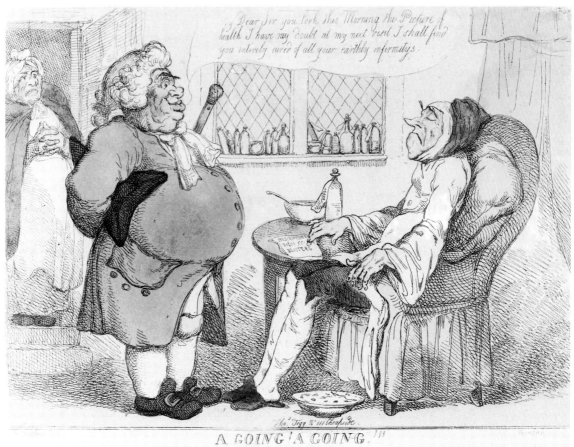

A GOING! A GOING.!!!

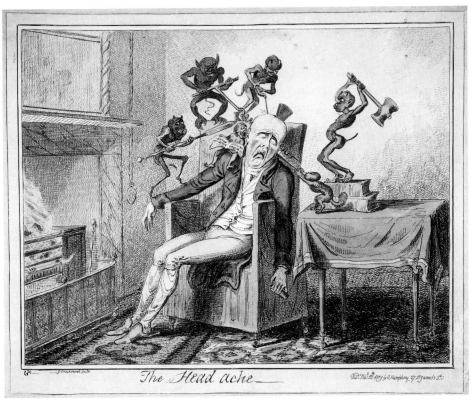

The Head ache

70

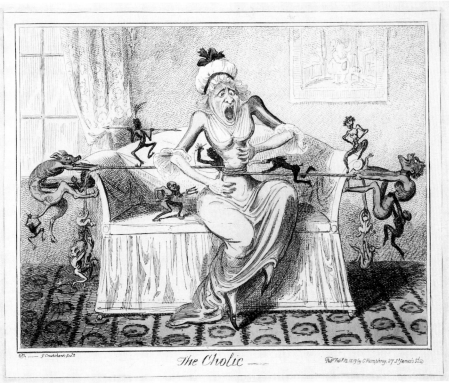

The Cholic

72

Hein, H., Pharmacy in Caricature, Frankfurt, 1964, no. 166

Lettered below scene:

"I have a secret art to cure / Each malady which men endure"

The scene, while a satire on the dubious nature of contemporary medicine, depicts in some detail the public interior of an early nineteenth century apothecary's shop. Indeed, 'APOTHECARIES HALL" appears on the lintel above the door to the street, from which enters a long queue of elderly and ill customers. A small 'Rowlandson' dog sits at lower left.

Behind the dispensing counter, beneath a large stuffed fish, and in front of an impressive display of shelves of carboys, wet and dry drug jars (all labelled with poisons: CANTHARI, ARSENIC, OPIUM, NITRE, VITRIOL), and a drug run, stands a fat apothecary. He is shown wearing an old-fashioned 'physical' wig, and concentrates on decanting a liquid into a medicine bottle via a funnel. More bottles, a mortar and pestle and a wet drug jar line the counter.

Two dispensary chairs at either end of the counter are occupied on the left by an aged and comatose woman, on the right by a fat John Bull, who, looking over his shoulder, starts in alarm at the appearance of the apothecary's assistant, a grinning skeleton, death, who (behind a curtain to the right and surrounded by much pharmaceutical equipment: sieves, syringes, saws, bottles and receivers), industriously pounds a large mortar marked: "SLOW.POISON".

PZ. 164

MARRYAT, Capt. Frederick (1792–1848)
etched by CRUIKSHANK, George (1792–1878)

70 The Head ache____

Pub^d. Feby. 12th 1819 by G. Humphrey 27 S^t. James's S^t.
[Marryat]
G Cruikshank fec^t

Etching hand coloured, 20.90 × 25.50 cm.
Prov.: Purchase 1956
Ref.: George, M. D., 9, 1949, no. 13439
        Zigrosser, C., Medicine and the Artist, New York, 1970, no. 87
        Cohn, A. M., 1924, no. 1186

A thin, elderly and bald man is slumped in an armchair by the fire grimacing in despair with upturned eyes, and holding a medicine bottle. He is tormented by six little demons who attack his head with auger, bit, mallet & wedge, and red-hot poker, one sings from a music-book in one ear, another blows a trumpet in his other.

Companion to "The Cholic", nos. 71 (PZ. 12), 72 (PZ. 11. 1–2).

PZ. 7. 1–4

MARRYAT, Capt. Frederick (1792–1848)
etched by CRUIKSHANK, George (1792–1878)

71 The Cholic――

Pub^d Feby. 12 1819 by G Humphrey, 27 St James's St.
[Marryat]
G Cruikshank fec^t.

Etching hand coloured, cut to 17.70 × 23.30 cm.
Prov.: Purchase 1956

First state.

An elderly woman, thin and haggard wearing cap and gown sits on a sofa screaming and writhing in agony as two naked demons haul tight a rope around her waist. Behind, on the wall is a picture of a fat woman in a bedroom drinking (gin?) from a decanter.

Companion to 'The Headache', no. 70 (PZ. 7).

PZ. 12

MARRYAT, Capt. Frederick (1792–1848)
etched by CRUIKSHANK, George (1792–1878)

72 The Cholic――

Pub^d Feby. 12 1819 by G Humphrey, 27 S^t. James's St.
[Marryat]
G Cruikshank fec^t.

Etching hand coloured, 20.00 × 25.00 cm.
WM: WHATMAN 1818
Ref.: George, M. D., 9, 1949, no. 13438

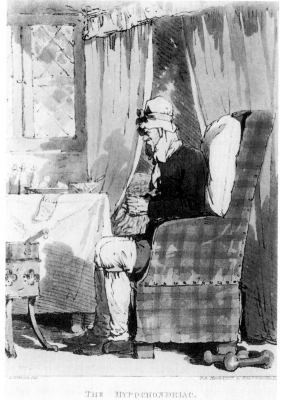

THE HYPOCHONDRIAC.

73

Second state of no. 71.

The second state has an additional 14 smaller demons, both heaving on the rope and tormenting the woman with trident, spear, whip and needle.

PZ. 11. 1–2

ATKINSON, John Augustus (1775–c.1833)

73 THE HYPOCHONDRIAC.
Pub. March 1. 1819. by Edwd. Orme Bond S^t.
A Atkinson Del

Etching and aquatint, cut to 25.00 × 18.50 cm.
Prov.: Purchase

Shows the patient, a typical image of the popular subject of the hypochondriac, huddled hands clasped and wrapped-up in coat, cap and gaiters, seated propped up with a pillow in an armchair before a table with his medicine bottles and prescription headed "PILLS", next to a portable gothick brazier with a steaming pan. A well-curtained bed is in the background.

PZ. 1

CRUIKSHANK, Isaac Robert (1789–1856), and CRUIKSHANK, George (1792–1878)

74 Jerry "beat to a standstill"! Dr Please'em's Prescription; Tom and Logic's condolence; and the "Slaveys" on the alert.
Pub^d. by Sherwood, Neely, Jones, Jany 1. 1822.
Drawn & Eng^d. by I. R. & G. Cruikshank

Etching and aquatint hand coloured, cut to 15.50 × 24.40 cm.
Prov.: Purchase 1960
Ref.: Pierce, E., Life in London, London, Sherwood, Neely & Jones, 1821, p. 361
George, M. D., 10, 1952, no. 14354
Cohn, A. M., 1924, no. 262

A bedroom scene in Corinthian House. An invalid Jerry is seated on a chair. Tom sits facing him holding a top-hat. The Doctor directed to the patient, an old nurse mixes gruel. In the background Logic, on a visit from the fleet, talks to the maid.

PZ. 17

SHERINGHAM, J.
etched by CRUIKSHANK, George (1792–1878)

75 Symptoms of Life in London or Love, Law, & Physic. __
Pub Augt. 28th 1821 by G Humphrey 27 St James's St London
J Sher^m. inv^t.
G Cruik fec^t.^d

Etching hand coloured, 26.00 × 38.70 cm.
WM: J WHATMAN TURKEY MILL
Prov.: Purchase

Ref.: George, M. D., 10, 1952, no. 14312A
Cohn, A. M., 1924, no. 1703

Second state.
Three designs side by side on one sheet.

(a) "CORDIALS & COMPOUNDS ... HODG[ES] BEST". Outside a druggists, locked and boarded for the night, a dandy is amused by two fashionable prostitutes who, unknown to him, are stealing his watch and wallet.

(b) Baliff and assistant apprehend a surprised dandy in the street.

(c) Sick room, the mantelpiece lined with medicine bottles, a thin, bald, doctor dressed in professional grey, with gold-topped cane and top-hat in hand, sits and studies his seated patient in nightshirt and cap. An old nurse stands behind the doctor.

The title is that of a farce by Kenney, first performed on 20th November 1812 at Covent Garden.

PZ. 22

MARRYAT, Capt. Frederick (1792–1848)
etched by CRUIKSHANK, George (1792–1878)

76 MIXING A RECIPE FOR CORNS __
Pub. by G. Humphrey 27 S^t. James's S^t. London Dec 4 1822
[Marryat]
G. C^k.

Etching hand coloured, cut to 19.50 × 24.00 cm.
Prov.: Purchase
Ref.: George, M. D., 10, 1952, no. 14443
Hein, H., Pharmacy in Caricature, Frankfurt, 1964, pp. 26–27
Cohn, A. M., 1924, no. 1740A

A satire on the trials of self-medication first published by Humphrey as the heading of a broadside "Recipe for Corns", 31 Mar 1819.

A sharp-faced old maid in spectacles, cap and petticoats sits in her bedroom, a scene of untidy and cluttered mayhem, by a fireplace lined with Delft tiles, as cats, lap-dogs, mice and parrot fight around her. Determinedly reading a clearly complicated recipe and mixing a pot on the roaring fire which spills over as she does so. By her chair is a table covered with medicine bottles, a mortar and pestle, packets, and raw ingredients, which also clutter the floor. On the far right is a curtained bed.

On the wall in the background is a case containing a glum, be-ribboned stuffed cat, and a picture of Suzanna suffering the advances of the Elders (from the Apocrypha, a woman accused of unchastity because she had refused male advances). The mantelpiece lintle is decorated with a burlesque scene of Diana, the virgin huntress, urging the hounds onto Actaeon. On the mantelpiece are peacock's feathers, bottles, spills, a mandarin figure, and a sea-shell.

PZ. 6

CRUIKSHANK, George (1792–1878)

77 The Blue Devils____!!
*Pub^d. by G. Humphrey 27 St James's St London – Jan^y.
10th. 1823 –
G. Cruikshank fec^t.*

Etching hand coloured, cut to 23.80 × 29.70 cm.
Trimmed to platemark.
WM: WHATMAN 1827
Prov.: Purchase 1956
Ref.: George, M. D., 10, 1952, no. 14598
      Cohn, A. M., 1924, no. 934

Second state.

A man, completely lost in depression, dressed in
nightgown, cap, breeches and slippers sits in a chair
close to a fireplace, empty save for a long bill. A number of small figures and devils torment him: a baliff
taps his shoulder and holds out a writ, a devil offers
him an open razor, a small figure tries to put a noose
around his neck. By his feet a miniature beadle leads
three pregnant women, an old-fashioned doctor hur-
ries towards him – followed by an undertaker with
a coffin. The pictures on the wall continue the theme
of misery, being shipwrecks, fires, and a picture of
himself being bullied by a woman.

Two books on a shelf, ''Buchans Domestic medicine'',
(see no. 85), and ''MISERIES of HUMAN LIFE (Folio)
VOL. 2222, PLATE XVIMD'', one book by the chair:
''ENNUI''.

PZ. 10

HEATH, William (1795–1840)

78 PAYING in KIND
*Pub may 12 1823 by G Humphrey 24 S^t. James S^t &
New Bond S^t.
WH-Del et sculp*

Etching hand coloured, 11.30 × 14.70 cm.
Ref.: George, M. D., 10, 1952, no. 14573

A foot-boy in livery, hat in hand, basket on arm has
brought a doctor's bill to a convalescent gentleman.
He sits in an armchair in a drawing room, wearing
a patterned nightgown and a cap and studies closely
through his spectacles, with some surprise, the very
long paper, saying (lettered in upper margin):

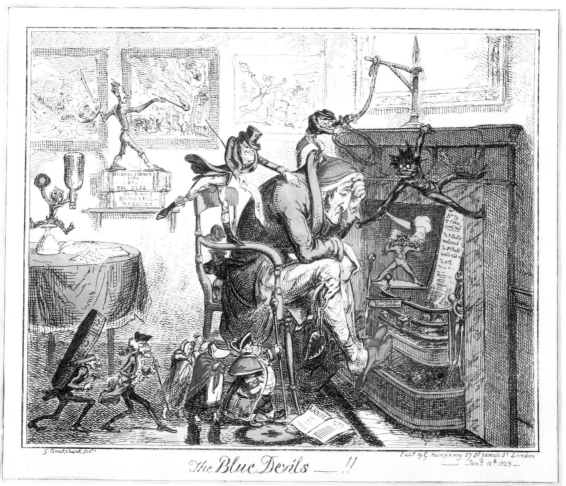

The Blue Devils ___!!

"Tell the Doctor I will certainly <u>pay</u> for the <u>Physic</u> but shall return the <u>Visits</u>!."

This charmingly executed satire, one of a set by Heath, alludes to the large sums charged by doctors' for visiting a patient, a lucrative practice forbidden to the rival apothecarys', who could only charge for the actual medicine.

PZ. 85

ANON.
etched by ROWLANDSON, Thomas
(1756–1827)

79 THE TOOTH ACHE, OR TORMENT & TORTURE.
PUBLISHED AUGUST 1,. 1823, BY JOHN FAIR-BURN, BROADWAY, LUDGATE HILL.
Rowlandson Scul. 1823

Etching hand coloured, 23.30 × 18.20 cm.
Prov.: Purchase 1972

A seated lady patient throws out her arms in alarm as a burly dentist probes her mouth with a stubby finger. By her side his boy assistant stands ready with a bowl and forceps, (behind him sits a 'Rowlandson' dog on stool). Beyond the counter an old woman with toothache enters, hanging in the background is a bird in cage and a pair of wigs on hooks.

A sign on background wall:

"BARNABY FACTOTUM. Draws Teeth. Bleeds & Shaves. WIGS made here, also Sausages. Wash Balls. black Puddings. Scotch Pills. Powder for the Itch. Red Herrings. Breeches Balls and small Beer by the maker IN UTRUMQUE PARATUS".

PZ. 180

ANON.

80 Sauntering down Bond Street, . . .
London, Published by W. Egerton, 1824.

Etching and aquatint hand coloured,
21.30 × 27.40 cm.
Prov.: Purchase
Ref.: Egerton, W., Day in the Life of a Sponge, London, 1824

Lettered below design:

"Sauntering down Bond Street, in the evening, to "Lose & neglect the creeping hours of time", espied an acquaintance on the opposite side of the way; was alive to the chance of a supper, darted across, when a heedless "Knight of the Whip", passing with his crazy vehicle, laid me senseless; thus conveyed to the shop of an Apothecary, was strip to ascertain where I was injured, "When sorrows come, they come not singly handed, but in battalions", had the mortification of being sufficiently sensible to be aware of the exposure of my wardrobe, without the power to prevent it, lost my supper, but gained a few bruises."

Scene in an Apothecary's study, in a room beyond can be seen the dispensery, counter with mortar and pestle, display cases with coloured, bottle and drug jars, and the street beyond. Four men undress the seated and helpless victim of a road accident, the concerned coachman looks on.

PZ. 45

FORRESTIER, Alfred Henry "CROWQUILL, Alfred" (1804–1872)
etched by CRUIKSHANK, George (1792–1878)

81 Indigestion.
Pub^d. Decr. 12th. 1825 by S Knight Sweetings alley, Royal Xchange
A Crowquill Esqr. del^t.
Etched by GC^k.

Etching hand coloured, cut to 17.00 × 23.00 cm.
Prov.: Purchase 1956
Ref.: George, M. D., 10, 1952, no. 14904
Cohn, A. M., 1924, no. 1233

A man, unshaven, pale and obviously in discomfort, sits facing between fire and window in an upper room. He wears a nightgown and slippers and holds his stomach with his hand while tormented by little figures and demons. One dangles a large pendulum, two tiny watchmen arrest a drunk.

A bottle of "Soda water" and a "plum pudding" are on the table, invitations to dinner are scattered at his feet. The books in the room are: "Black Draught" and "Essay on Digestion". The full moon seen through window disturbingly resembles a pudding.

Companion to 'Jealousy', no. 120 (PZ. 8).

PZ. 16, 1–3

HEATH, Henry (fl. 1824–1850)

82 REDUCTION.
Arithmetic Plate, 5th.
Pub^d July, 1827, by William Cole, Newgate Street,
Drawn & Etched by HHeath.

Etching hand coloured, 17.00 × 22.00 cm.
Prov.: Purchase 1957

A satire on one of the many health 'cures' fashionable during the nineteenth century (see also no. 92). On the left, several healthy but fat patients await the attentions of the busy operator of a "STOMACH PUMP.", who is energetically pumping out a fat man seated in a chair, the contents pour in a tin tub near two tiny, reduced animals. On the right an unhappy, but very thin man feels his flaccid belly. On the wall is a picture of a very large and a very thin dog captioned: "specimen of the Reduction of a Dog Performed by the Stomach-Pump in 3 Operations."

PZ. 79

ANON.

83 Devils at home – breathing a vein
[n.d.]

Etching, cut to 13.50 × 20.70 cm. (PZ. 156), hand coloured, cut to 7.90 × 10.00 cm. (PZ. 157)
WM: [W]HATMAN 1827 (PZ. 157)

Coloured (PZ. 157) and uncoloured, impressions.

Three naked, cloven-hoofed devils watch anxiously as a larger, tusked and bearded devil, an open lancet on the ground by his hooves, bleeds a fourth lying between them.

PZ. 156
PZ. 157

CRUIKSHANK, Isaac Robert (1789–1856)
cut by "GW"

84 ROBERT CRUIKSHANK'S RANDOM SHOTS. – (Nº. 2.) A CHOLERA PATIENT.
Published by TOMLINSON, 24, Great Newport Street, [n.d.]
Robᵗ. Cruikshank
GW

Woodcut, cut to 25.10 × 23.40 cm.
Prov.: Purchase

A worried and emaciated man dressed in rags sits on a stool marked "STARVATION" next to a trestle resting on bones labelled "BOARD OF HEALTH", he holds a massive pill in his left hand, his right elbow rests on a box "Blue Pills" on the table. Also on the table is a large, anthropomorphic-medicine bottle with claw-like hands marked "Emetic", with a label "The dose to be repeated", around which dance a ring of tiny devils. Below the table squats a skull-headed bird bearing the words "Fee Fo Fum".

PZ. 25

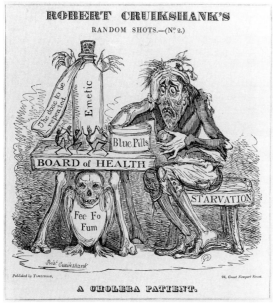

84

DAGLEY, Richard (c. 1765–1841)
etched by BROOKE, William Henry (1772–1860)

85 TAKING PHYSIC
London, Published by John Warren, Old Bond St, W. B. Whittaker, Ave Maria La[ne] [n.d.]
R. Dagley del.
W H Brooke sculp

Etching, cut to 12.00 × 9.50 cm.

A man seated in front of a screen, wearing cap and nightgown with dishevelled stockings, turns his head away and throws up his arms in horror from a nurse in gown and cap pouring medicine into a bowl. Next to his chair is a table with a spitoon, a medicine bottle, spoon, and a copy of "BUCHAN" (Buchan, W. *Domestic Medicine; or, the Family Physician: being an attempt to render the Medical Art more generally useful, by shewing people what is in their own power both with respect to the Prevention and Cure of Diseases, chiefly calculated to recommend a proper attention to Regimen and Simple Medicines.* Edinburgh, 1769. Nineteen editions of this immensely popular work were sold during the author's lifetime and it continued to be produced until well into the nineteenth century.)

PZ. 42

ANON.

86 Advice gratis.
[n.d. c. 1830?]

Etching hand coloured, cut to 27.00 × 26.50 cm.
Prov.: Purchase 1977

Interior of a chemist and druggists shop, with carboys displayed in the window, and on the glass panels of the door: "ADVICE GRATIS FROM 10 TILL 2". An unhappy customer, an old woman a crutch under one arm, and carrying a basket full of medicine bottles, remonstrates with the druggist:

"Seven shillings! Lork sir, I thought it was gratis!!!"

The satisfied druggist replies:

"Aye my good woman we give the advice, but charge for the medicine."

Behind them is the counter with a pill tile and a mortar and pestle, behind the counter a drug run and drug jars.

PZ. 176

ANON.

87 A CURE FOR A COLD
Tregears Flights of Humor no 32.
Published by G. Tregear 123 Cheapside London 1833.

Lithograph coloured, 20.00 × 8.00 cm.
Prov.: Purchase 1955

Lettered below scene:

"HERE'S A GO; I MUST KEEP MY FEET IN HOT-WATER 20 MINUTES TAKE TWO QUARTS OF

GRUEL WRAP MY HEAD IN FLANEL AND TAL-
LOW MY NOSE."

A man, in hopeless misery, sits in an armchair wearing a large overcoat over his nightshirt, a muffler and
a cap. With his left hand he stirs a bowl of gruel on
a nearby table, his feet are immersed in a tub of steaming water. A satire on the complicated and incongruous remedies for even the simplest of maladies.

PZ. 86

COURCELL, A.

88 PAIN.
[n.d.]
A Courcell Fecit

Etching and aquatint hand coloured, cut to
15.20 × 13.00 cm.

A three-quarter length portrait of a seated man, wearing cap, nightgown over shirt and breeches. He
prepares, with deep disgust, to drink a cup of medicine which he holds in his right hand, a medicine bottle labelled "to be Taken Immediately" in his left,
the arm resting on a table having a pillbox marked
"Pills one Morning & Night" and a bottle "one fourth
to be taken every hour".

This image is almost identical to no. 90 (PZ. 168), and
no. 89 (PZ. 158), and is probably derived from no. 56
(PZ. 50), 'Taking Physic'.

PZ. 29

ANON.

89 [Untitled]
[n.d. c. 1835?]
Signed in pencil on mount: Taking physic

Watercolour and gouache 13.90 × 11.50 cm.

This is an identical, smaller, and reversed version of
'En gouterai-je?', no. 90 (PZ. 168), and might possibly
even be a finished preliminary watercolour for the
lithograph.

PZ. 158

NOËL, Leon
lithographed by NOËL, F.

90 En gouterai-je?.
*Publié par Giraldon-Bovinet et Comp^{im}., M^{dm}.
d'estampes, Coumessconndires, rue Pavée, St André, N°.
5. [n.d. c. 1835]*
L Noël
Lithog de F. Noël

Lithograph coloured, 35.00 × 28.50 cm.
Prov.: Purchase 1977

A man in an armchair, wearing the usual cap and a
nightgown over a shirt and tie, stirs a cup of medicine, a look of revulsion on his face. On a small table
is an open book and a medicine bottle.

See also no. 89 (PZ. 158), above.

PZ. 168

ANON. "~"

91 THE CONSUMPTIVE PATIENT
Funny characters No 7.
London W Spooner 377 Strand. [n.d. c. 1835]
~ delt.

Lithograph coloured, 26.00 × 20.00 cm.
Prov.: Purchase 1956

Lettered below design:

"Please Doctor I've brought the little boy wot's going
into a decline!"

The doctor pauses in his reading of "The Times
advertisements" to regard a woman who speaks to
him, and an overdressed, obese and repulsive child.
The walls have shelves of jars containing anatomical
specimens, a diploma, and a large pestle and mortar.

PZ. 146

ANON.

92 THE MUMMY STATE.
PLATE, II.
[Messrs. Fores, 41 Picadilly, corner of Sackville Street]
[n.d. c. 1822–41]

Etching hand coloured, 12.10 × 21.00 cm.
Ref.: The Sure Water Cure, or Hydropathist,
London, [n.d.], pl. 11

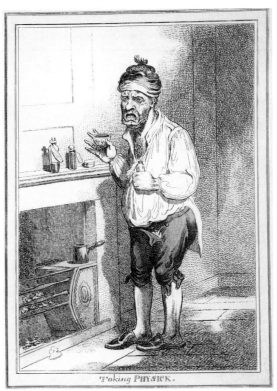
Taking PHYSICK.

93

Lettered on facing page:

"The patient having been made a client of (Vulgo
stript of every thing; common sense not excluded.)
is tightly enveloped in blankets to perspire if he lives
long enough, he is usually made a Mummy of or
cured, the chances are equal, the hands being confined, water is given plentifully through a tube,
obviously those who thus expect to be cured, will
suck in any thing, any quantity, and at any price!"

Two quacks and an assistant attend to a patient
undergoing water therapy. The patient, at the end
of a fire pump, fire buckets on shelf behind, camp
bed, watering can, tubs.

One of the "Amusing Works" published by the Fores
in the 1820s–40s. It professes to advocate the current
craze, the home water cure, against the "idle sneerer
at novelties".

49207

GILLRAY, James (1756–1815)
engraved by ANON.

93 Taking PHYSIC.
London Published by John Miller, Bridge Street & W.

Blackwood, Edinburgh
[n.d. c. 1850]

Engraving hand coloured, 35.00 × 27.50 cm.
Prov.: Purchase 1955

Late copy of no. 56.

PZ. 49

LAGUILLERMIE, Frederic Auguste (b. 1841
fl. 1863–1923), and RAINAUD

**94 Le médecin à la Maison ou conseils utiles pour
secourir les Blessés et guérir tous les Accidens [sic]**
Maison Basset, 33 rue de Seine, Paris [n.d. c. 1870?]
Compose et Gravé par Laguillermie et Rainaud

Etching hand coloured, cut to 53.30 × 70.20 cm.

[The Doctor at Home or useful advice for assisting
the injured and recovering from all Accidents.]

Illustrations of twenty-four domestic health prob-
lems, including "Douleurs des Dents", "Mal der
Mer", "Maladies des Yeux", "Hemorrages", "Indi-
gestions", and "Contre Poisons", with suggested
remedies.

PZ. 187

ADVERTISEMENTS AND PROPRIETARIES

As a subject of widespread popular concern at
this period, the lucrative trade in proprietary
medicines lent itself to the art of caricature,
both as a source of satire and, increasingly, as
a form of advertisement and promotion. Arising
from a tradition of the itinerant seller of medicines, these were sold on the basis of their capa-
city to cure almost every conceivable medical
condition. By the 19th century some of the most
famous products had created great fortunes for
their purveyors and inventors. In certain cases
entrepreneurial businessmen, outside the medical or pharmaceutical profession, such as William Rowland, the wholesale perfumer,
proprietor of Rowland's Macassar Oil (97), and
James Morison (var. Morrison, Morisson), of
the infamous vegetable pills (100). In the case
of the latter, much of the success of this product
arose from the convincing espousal of an alternative, though bogus, medical philosophy.
Other products were associated with members
of the medical establishment such as Dr James
of his eponymous powders or Dr Perkins,
inventor of the metallic tractors (96).

These products played an important part in
shaping popular ideas about medical treatment,
finding a lucrative source of custom in a
demand for medical panaceas, cures and
remedies. According to the countless
testimonials in the advertising for certain products, they attracted sales from patients either
unable to afford or disillusioned with conventional medical treatment. An alternative form
of endorsement was that which received sanc-
tion from respectable medical authority (110).
Either way, the proselytising promotion of
these products was often filled with unsubstan-
tiated claims as well as erroneous medical explanation and terminology.

From the 18th century the sale of these products expanded dramatically, aided by the use
of the printed advertisement and their sale
through booksellers and stationers (106, 107,
108). Gradually, however, the chemist and
druggist came to recognise the financial value
of this business and thus developed a role in
their marketing. Hence, one of the most familiar
ways in which the pharmacist is depicted in
comic images is advising the customer about the
benefits of a particular product.

ANON. "ROUGHSCRATCH, Titian Angelo"
by "WOODCUTTER, Raphael"

95 The Magazine's Blown Up
*Publish'd according to Act of Parliament For J Cook
in, Pater Noster Row, [n.d. c. 1770]*

Raphael Woobcutter S[c] [sic]
Titian Angelo Roughscratch invt

Woodcut, cut to 15.00 × 11.00 cm.
Prov.: Purchase

A signboard outside a brick town building announces: "Dr. JAMES'S POWDER SOLD HERE", a sign in the window advertises: "BRITISH OIL". Outside, a man stands by papers lettered "THE OLD WOMANS MAG", "LADYS MAG", "UNIVERSAL MAG", "GRAND MAG OF MAG", "MAGAZINE OF MAGAZINE", "STUDENT", "KAPELION", which are engulfed in flames from a commode, the true storehouse of the forementioned paper, marked "THE JAKES OF GENIUS".

This crudely executed satire would appear to be directed against a rival publisher and bookseller John Newbery (1713–1767), the sole agent for Dr. James's Fever Powder. This cure-all, patented in 1747 by Dr Robert James (fl. 1750), was an antimonial and mercurial preparation which continued in use until the twentieth century. Its' continued popularity owed much to clever advertising by James and particularly by Newbery, who allegedly collaborated with Oliver Goldsmith (c. 1730–1774), in the writing of the famous children's book 'Goody Two Shoes', where not surprisingly one finds the child's father died 'seized with a violent fever in a place where Dr James's Powder was not to be had'. Ironically, Goldsmith's premature death was said to be as a result of dosing himself with James's Powders against the advice of his doctors (see also no. 26).

PZ. 133

GILLRAY, James (1756–1815)

96 METALIC TRACTORS.
[Humphrey H,] [11th November 1801]
Jas Gillray del

Etching and aquatint hand coloured, cut to 17.80 × 21.60 cm.
Prov.: Donation 1945, Wyatt
Ref.: George, M. D., 8, 1947, no. 9761
 Hein, H., Pharmacy in Caricature, Frankfurt, 1964, p. 118
 Wright, T., The Works of James Gillray the Caricaturist, London, [n.d.] p. 281
 Holländer, E., Die Karikatur und Satire in der Medezin, Stuttgart, 1921, pl. 8

A thin man, his hair powdered and in a long queue, holds one tractor in his mouth as he applies the second tractor to the carbuncled nose of a seated John Bull, from which bursts sheets of flame as the stunned John's physical wig falls off. His bemused dog looks on. Picture on wall of Bacchus astride a barrel.

On a nearby table is a newspaper, beneath a clay pipe with a steaming jug and a bottle of "BRANDY", a bowl of sugar with tongs, a half lemon and a goblet with a spoon. The paper headed: "The True Briton", is lettered:

"Theatre Dead Alive . . . / Grand Exhibition in Leicester Square / just arrived from America the Rod of Esculapius / Perkinism in all its Glory being a certain cure for all Disorders Red Noses Gouty Toes Windy Bowls Broken Legs HumpBacks / just Discover'd the Grand Secret of the Philosp[] Stone with the true way of turning all metal into Gold pro bono publico"

Perkins metallic tractors, patented in 1798 by the American Elisha Perkins, who unfortunately died of Yellow Fever in New York the following year while demonstrating his cure for the disease. The Tractors had only to be regularly drawn across the affected area of the body for a cure to be achieved through electricity. His son brought the invention to Britain, where the craze for the Tractors was such that even a 'Perkinean Institution' was established, for the free treatment of the poor who could not afford the price of five guineas for a pair of the miraculous Tractors. Perkins eventually returned to America with a fortune said to be £10,000.

PZ. 60

ROWLANDSON, Thomas (1756–1827)

97 MACASSAR OIL, An Oily Puff for Soft Heads.
[T. Tegg 111 Cheapside 15th May 1814]
Rowlandson Del

Etching hand coloured, cut to 33.50 × 23.50 cm.
Prov.: Purchase 1956
Ref.: George, M. D., 9, 1949, no. 12405
 Hein, H., Pharmacy in Caricature, Frankfurt, 1964, no. 52
 Holländer, E., Die Karikatur und Satire in der Medezin, Stuttgart, 1921, p. 307

Lettered upper right corner:

"Macassar Oil for the Growth of Hair is the finest invention ever known for increasing hair on bald Places, Its virtues are pre-eminent for improving and beautifying the Hair of Ladies and Gentlemen__This invaluable Oil recommended on the basis of truth and experience is sold at One Guinea Pr Bottle by all the Perfumers and Medicine Vendors in the Kingdom".

In the corner of a room lined with shelves of bottles: "Wig Oil One Guinea Pr Bottle" and a large jar with a mug placed on its lip; a perfumer, in apron and cap, stands beside a fat man seated in a chair above a wide-brimmed bowl and applies the latest quack remedy of Macassar or Rowlands oil to his bald head from a straw-covered bottle. On the floor next to the man is his tall "FOOLS CAP" with asses ears. Behind a fat lady regards her upright hair with some surprise in a mirror below a notice:

"Wonderful Discovery carroty or Grey Whiskers changed to Black Brown or Blue____"

PZ. 181

GILLRAY, JAMES (1756–1815)
etched by CRUIKSHANK, George (1792–1878)

98 a Cure for Drowsiness__or____A PINCH OF CEPHALIC
{__Pubd. Jany. 25th. 1822 by G Humphrey 27 St. James's St. London__
Etched by G Cruickshank from a sketch by the late Jas. Gillray}

Etching hand coloured, cut to 26.00 × 20.00 cm.
Ref.: George, M. D., 10, 1952, no. 14442
Cohn A. M., 1924, no. 1031

A stout man sits facing in a chair by a fireplace and sneezes violently, startling a small dog at his feet, having taken some cephalic snuff from a small box in his left hand in a desperate attempt to continue his study of the tedious "Parliamentry Debates" resting on his knee. To the right is a small table with a clay pipe on a stand, a glass decanter and a large, steaming, glass cup and spoon. On the mantelpiece is an oriental squatting figure and a bust of "Morpheus", the god of sleep. Cruikshank etched this from a design of Gillray and included an oval portrait of him on the wall in the background. Cephalic snuff was taken especially as a remedy for colds.

PZ. 192

GRANT, Charles Jameson (fl. 1828–1846)

99 Morsels of Mirth Nᵒ 2
Printed by L. M. Lefevre, Newman St.
C J Grant invᵗ & [−]

Lithograph coloured, 49.50 × 39.00 cm.
Purchase 1958

See following description, no. 100 (PZ. 175).

PZ. 47

GRANT, Charles Jameson (fl. 1828–1846)

100 EXTRAORDINARY EFFECTS OF THE VEGETABLE PILLS ON A TAILOR, WHO HAVING CABBAGED TO A GREAT EXTENT, WAS TAKEN ILL & AFTER SWALLOWING 130 BOXES OF THE AFORESAID PILLS, PRESENTE [sic] THE ABOVE PHENOMENON..
[n.d. c. 1830–40]

Lithograph coloured, cut to 35.00 × 30.00 cm.
Prov.: Purchase 1977

Scene in a bedroom, an old woman in cap, spectacles and apron with large knife stands in front of a man in cap and nightgown in chair who looks aghast at the cabbage sprouting from his nose. Her speech balloon has been obliterated. Design included as part of no. 99 (PZ. 47), with eight smaller vignettes.

PZ. 175

ANON.

101 [Untitled]
[n.d. c. 1830–40]

Lithograph coloured, cut to 16.80 × 12.10 cm.
Prov.: Purchase 1956

Lettered below design:

"Mercutio: He has made worms meat of me – go for a Surgeon – Spectator: Let me advise you to try these Morrisons Pills No2 – take 10 the first Dose – repeat it every ten minutes"

An actor as Mercutio lies dying, but a concerned spectator leans forward out of his stage box, he wears spectacles and holds a pillbox in his hand. Morison's Pills came in two strengths, No. 1 which was a mild aperient, and the stronger purgative No. 2.

PZ. 125

ANON.

102 UNIVERSAL PILLS Nᵒ1.
London W Spooner 377 Strand. [n.d. c. 1830–40]

Lithograph coloured, 24.80 × 20.80 cm.
Prov.: Purchase

A black servant in extremely rich livery and carrying a staff of office is a customer in a chemists and druggists, the walls are covered with posters: "MORRISONS PILLS WARRENTED TO EFFECT A CHANGE IN 24 HOURS", "PILLS for the NORTH POLE", and behind the counter are shelves of "TESTIMONIALS"; he asks the bald and bespectacled man behind the counter:

"Massa Doctor, you tink I get more rite for taking you Pills?"

"Decidedly Sir! about two thousand boxes more will without doubt render you as white as a Lily!"

PZ. 135

ANON.

103 UNIVERSAL PILLS Nᵒ2.
W Spooner 377 Strand. [n.d. c. 1830–40]

Lithograph coloured, 37.75 × 31.25 cm.
Prov.: Purchase
Ref.: Hein, H., Pharmacy in Caricature, Frankfurt, 1964, no. 63

A tall young man is in conversation with a short, old-fashioned chemist pounding a mortar at his counter, behind the counter are shop rounds and a drug run, the chemist looks up from his work:

"What d'ye say, your Father's confined too? Bless me, why don't he try Morrison's Pills?"

"Cos I dont think he knowd as they vos good things to get him out of Vitecross Street Prisun!"

PZ. 136

ANON.

104 UNIVERSAL PILLS Nᵒ 3.
W Spooner 377 Strand. [n.d. c. 1830–40]

Lithograph coloured, 31.25 × 24.00 cm.
Prov.: Purchase 1956

"This here Board is a hexact representation of me as I vos afore I took to Morrisons Pills and only took 480 Boxes!! I lived on nothink else for a vortnight."

A man, wearing a top-hat, and so obese he is bursting out of his clothes, carries an advertising board for Morison's pills showing his skeletal appearance before he began his treatment.

PZ. 137

ANON.

105 UNIVERSAL PILLS N° 4,
W Spooner 377 Strand. (n.d. c. 1830–40]

Lithograph coloured, 39.75 × 28.50 cm.
Prov.: Purchase

"Here's a precious go them hinfernal vegatable pills have taken root in my nose. It was reddish before but now it's carotty!"

A man in shirtsleeves and cap stands directed to the right looking at himself in a dressing-table mirror. His nose has turned into an enormous carrot as a result of taking Morison's Pills.

PZ. 138

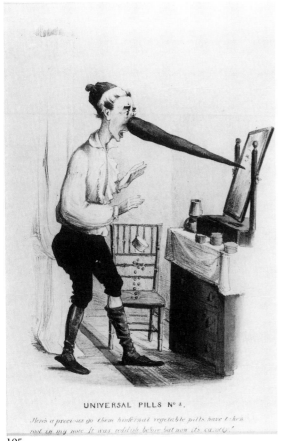

UNIVERSAL PILLS N° 4.

Here's a precious go them hinfernal vegetable pills have taken root in my nose. It was reddish before but now its carotty.

105

ANON.

106 HODGSONS GENUINE PATENT MEDICINES / Dʳ. JAMES'S ANTIBILIOUS PILLS
London Pubᵈ by O Hodgson 111 Fleet Street [n.d. c. 1830–40]

Etching hand coloured, cut to 39.00 × 32.00 cm.
Prov.: Purchase 1977

Lettered below design:

"Betty, what have you done with the PILLS I bought this morning? O marm, you said they was for the BILE so I put em into the copper but I don't think they will make the clothes a good colour".

A well dressed woman wearing a large ribboned bonnet is in conversation with her servant.

PZ. 165

ANON.

107 HODGSONS GENUINE PATENT MEDICINES / CURE FOR THE ITCH
[Hodgson] *Pubᵈ. 111 Fleet Street* [n.d. c. 1830–40]

Etching hand coloured, cut to 39.00 × 32.00 cm.
Prov.: Purchase 1977

Lettered below design:

"I hear Sir you are famous for Doctoring the Scotch Fiddle, so I have brought you this, it was bought in Edenboro and [ha]s got a little out of order, you see, coming over on the Steamer".

A fiddle-player in patched clothes presents a surprised chemist with a broken fiddle. The Scotch Fiddle was a colloquial term for venereal disease.

PZ. 166

ANON.

108 HODGSON'S GENUINE PATENT MEDICINES 1 / INFANTS PRESERVATIVE
[Hodgson] *Pubᵈ. 111 Fleet Street* [n.d. c. 1830–40]

Etching hand coloured, cut to 39.00 × 32.00 cm.
Prov.: Purchase 1977

Lettered below design:

"O Mʳˢ. Easy, your house says it's going to tumble down upon the spot and your Child is in the cockloft".
"Never you mind Miss Fume, I gave it a bottle of Infants Preservative before I came out so there is no danger".

Two women, one a pauper dressed in rags, the other in her working clothes discuss the state of the tumble-down tenement in the background.

PZ. 167

ANON.

109 MORISON'S PILLS / THE TRUE LIFEPRESERVER.

London Pub^d by O Hodgson 111 fleet Street [n.d. c. 1838]

Lithograph coloured, 28.00 × 40.90 cm.
Prov.: Purchase 1983

A sailor in land rig, with long pigtail and tar hat sits jauntily astride a large crate full of "MORRISON" pillboxes and marked: "MORRISONS PILLS For SEA SERVICE". He smokes a long clay pipe, in front of him are a glass of rum and a ?queue of tobacco?, and says:

"You Swabs may crack about your Life preservers in fair weather; but when a bit of a breeze springs up Lord bless you any body can see its all flam".

Around him others, personifications of various famous proprietary medicines, flounder in the waves. They include a Friar who clings to a huge bottle of "FRIARS BALSAM", two men wearing "Life preservers" holding on to a crate marked "COLLEGE OF HEALTH" containing ducks which "Quack", a widow Welch who falls from a capsized boat, "CON-STITUTION", a Quaker, and a man with "GOUT pills".

PZ. 173

CRUIKSHANK, George (1792–1878)

110 The FOX and the GOOSE.
Designed Etched & Published by George Cruikshank 1833

Etching, 18.80 × 27.90 cm.
Prov.: Purchase

Below scenes the text composed of several doggerel verses:

"A Fox there is who has such Knowledge
that his Dwelling House he calls a "COLLEGE"
And Geese flock to him from all quarters
Bringing Wives & Sons & Daughters
He tells the Geese, that their ills he's able
To cure with his Pills of Vegetable

He makes Goose hay his 'COLLEGE' rent
And calls himself the 'President'!

And so Goose thinks he can; good lack!
For 'Cackle' hath great faith in 'Quack' –
So he lives on Goose each day I ween,
His House is built on 'Ganders Green',
His Carriage wheels on 'Goose Grease' turn,
He fat of Goose for oil doth burn.

And not in trifles over nice,
'Tis he himself enacts the 'Vice'!!

He plucks their feathers for his bed,
On Down of Goose he lays his head,
He gets his Goose & eke his Stuffing
By Cramming Geese with Pills & Puffing;
He writes his Puffs with 'Grey Goose quill',
Of 'Goose = berry = fool' he has his fill,

And tho' 'tis strange 'tis also true
He is himself the 'Members' too!!!"

Another 'COLLEGE' there is I ween
Which may in Newman Street be seen

And there two Foxes, 'Charles & John'
Carry the very same system on – !"

A central vignette flanked by two smaller on either side. In the main a fox, dressed in a frock coat, and standing on a box of Morison's Universal Vegetable Pills addresses a flock of eagerly attentive geese. Saying:

"My 'Universal Pills' are quite divine!
If one don't do, you may take nine."

Behind him is the front of a building titled: "BRITISH COLLEGE OF HEALTH ESTABLISHED 1828", and over the street is the "LONDON COLLEGE OF HEALTH", and a smaller flock of geese gather around its porch on which two more foxes display medicines and pillboxes.

The smaller scenes have a fox dressed in the manner of an 18th century doctor offering a box of pills to a goose in a lady's cap. A fox addressing a flock of geese by a tree, a fox outside his shop "J.FOX Poulterer" serving a dressed goose to a goose, and a fox drummer leading a file of goose-stepping geese.

The British College of Health was established in 1828 by Morison and was used to defend his system of medicine and promote his pills. It is one of the accurately rendered buildings in the background, the other is the rival London College of Health, managed by physicians.

PZ. 15

GRANT, Charles Jameson (fl. 1828–1846)

111 EXTRAORDINARY EFFECTS OF MORRISONS VEGETABLE PILLS!
Grant's Oddities N° 1
Author of Tegear's Flights of Humour [– –] / *London pub by J Kendrick, 54 Leicester Squ^r. & where may be had a great Variety of Cheap Books Caricatures Album Scraps, Prints &c &c / NB Now Publishing a Comic Frontispiece / The Comic Almanac for 1834, Price 3^d* [– – –] *N° 1 / of Every Body's Album & Caricature Magazine. / Jany 10th 1834*
CJG Invent & Del.

Lithograph coloured, 33.50 × 27.50 cm.
Prov.: Purchase

Lettered below design:

"Vy Snook is that you ! Vell if I arnt completely Struck! Vy Ven did you change your Vooden Legs for Cork'uns!__? Cork ones! now do they look like a Pair of Cork ones. No old Boy they are real Flesh and Blood, and ten times a Better Pair than wot I was Born with, it'll only cost you a Shilling my tulip, and you'll have as good a Pair of Stumps as myself Yesterday you must know I bought a Box of Mor-risons Uniwersal Wegetable Pills, for a Swelling in my Thighs, well, so I took'em all afore I went to Bed and when I awakes in the morning to kick of the

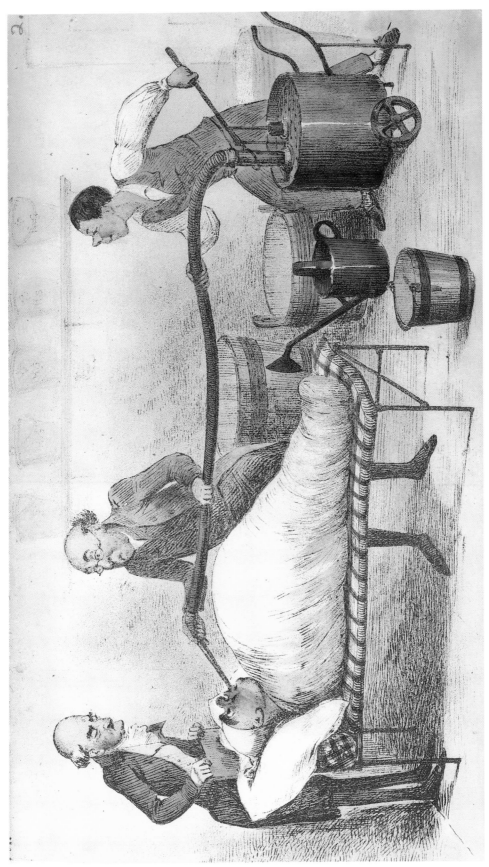

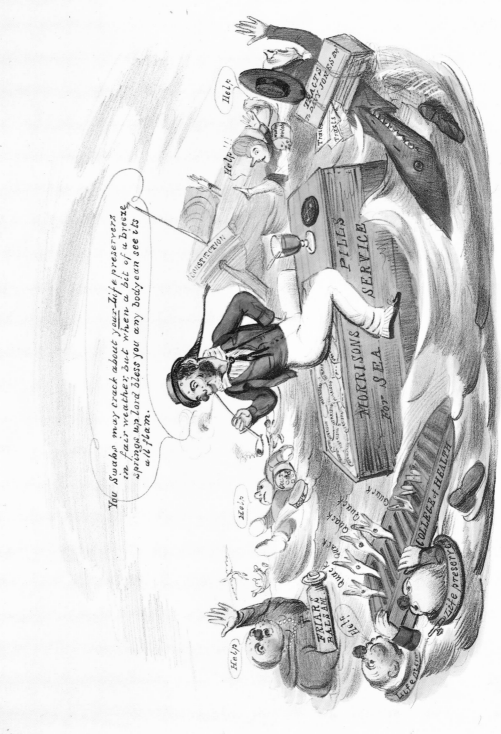

MORISON'S PILLS

THE TRUE LIFE PRESERVER.

109

clothes. I'm bless'd if I did'nt find myself with these'ere Couple of Jolly good Legs and my Old Wooden ones right at the bottom of the Bed!!!"

Two ragged friends meet, the one on the left proudly showing his new legs, his wooden legs under his arm, his legless companion on the right regarding him with amazement.

PZ. 59

GRANT, Charles Jameson (fl. 1828–1846)

112 **Awful effects of morison's vegetable pills !!!!!!**
LONDON Printed & Pub^d by T Davison N° 11 Paternoster Row Novr 5th 1835
C J Grant, Inv^t Del

Lithograph coloured, cut to 22.00 × 23.50 cm.
Prov.: Purchase

Lettered below design:

"Oh! Lawk a daisy me! Look here sir! Why you are cover'd all over with Grass!!—I shoud'nt at all wonder if it isn't taking so many of them Wegetable pills. They have no doubt taken root in your inside, & you sitting so long by the fire have made 'em Wegetate thro' your skin!!

This Print must be exposed to a gentle heat before the fire"

PZ. 74

ANON.

113 **[Untitled]**
Pubd 1836, by. G. S. Tregear, Cheapside.

Lithograph coloured, cut to 20.50 × 30.20 cm.
Prov.: Purchase

Two agricultural workmen in boots, breeches, smocks and neckchiefs in a cottage garden, one has entered from the gate on the left, he stands scratching his head, a pitchfork over his shoulder:

"Whoy Robin lad, wot be'st thee at?"

His companion kneels by a bed of worm-eaten cabbages on which he drops pills:

"Whoy these Cabbage's be Eaten nearly all up, and I be zowing zum o' them <u>Wegitable Pills</u>, they cure'd I o' the <u>Worms</u>, zo I means to try what em'll do for the <u>Cabbage's</u>". [sic]

PZ. 149

ANON.

114 **ADVICE (to Costermongers) GRATIS.**
[Tregear, Cheapside] [n.d. c. 1830–40]

Lithograph coloured, cut to 24.00 × 22.00 cm.
Prov.: Purchase

"How to set up in Business, Give your Hanimal a feed of Morrissons Wegetable Pills. and you will have no occasion to go to Common Garden blow me!!!"

A working man accurately depicted in the distinctive dress of a coster (see Mayhew, H., Life and Labour of the London Poor, 1851–62), of breeches, short jacket and cap, and smoking a short pipe is shown riding a donkey (the illustration is an accurate depiction of the proper donkey seat), which sprouts abundant carrots, turnips, and cabbages. The title is a pun on the free medical advice that chemists and druggists offered to customers.

PZ. 134

SALA, George Augustus (1828–1896)

115 **The Arts and Manufactures of the Medical Profession and the Marvels of the British College of Health.**
[c. 1845–50]

Etching hand coloured, cut to 6.40 × 21.70 cm.
Ref.: Anon., The Great Exhibition "Wot is To Be" . . . , Published by the Committee of the Society for keeping things in their place, London, 1850.

Part of the panorama only, two sobbing doctors, dressed in grey, titled: "Members of the Colleges of Surgeons and Physicians lamenting the———downfall of the Guinea Trade"

A man carrying a very large composition mortar and pestle, titled: "Disconsolate Apothecary with pestle and mortar reversed"

A man with a huge prescription: "Ars. alb, Nux. vom., Merc. & prus. ac.", captioned: "A real prescription, Price £1/1. Expected in a few years, to be as valuable for its rarity as any Manuscript in the British Museum".

A man carrying a long tray of poison bottles: "Prize specimens of the stock in trade of Doctors Shops." labelled, "Arsenic", "Nux Vomica", "Prussic Acid", "Opium", and "Morphine".

PZ. 57

CONCEPTS AND EMOTIONS

Among some of the most accomplished caricatures are those which illustrate abstract ideas. Familiar situations, often comic in content, are the subject of images entitled with concepts or conditions such as envy, jealousy and greed (116). In the classic tradition of caricature, the object of these prints is to convey the corruption of moral values and the basic weakness of human instinct, though their subject is likely to be a universal theme of behaviour or experience in contrast to those which relate to specific characters or scenes of known social or political significance. On occasion, the caricaturists' technique, often dependant on a recognisable battery of both the literal and metaphoric imagery, lends itself with considerable success and originality to this form.

The use of medical or pharmaceutical imagery is employed in a group of these images, even when the subject has little to do with these subjects. It can provide not only the ministering figure of the physician, apothecary or pharmacist but the paraphernalia of medication for great comic effect. The notion of punishment for a human vice, weakness or misdemeanour is a common idea, and one often expressed through the metaphor of medication. Portrayed as a penance, some images show that the administration of highly unpalatable medicine can deliver the victim from self-inflicted suffering while, in others, it is depicted as the medium of retribution. The most straightforward satires are those which illustrate the physical perils of excess, especially the dangerous consequences of drink. But medicine is also revealed as a more general source of unpleasant and punitive associations, even as a treatment for sins of a moral character.

PATERRE
etched by FILLOEUL

116 LE GLOUTON
a Paris chez Filloeul à l'entrée de la rüe du Fouarre au batiment neuf, par la rüe Galande. A.P.D.R.
Paterre pinxit.
Filloeul Sculp 1736

Etching and engraving hand coloured, cut to 32.80 × 36.30 cm.

Lettered below design:

Un Glouton opulent, qui faison ses delices
De remplir a grands frais son ventre spacieux,
Et de voir entasser à differents services
Sur sa table des mets friands et precieux,
Ordonne qua souper pour lui seul on appreste
Un Elurgeon auguel on note que la teste.

Il soupe; mais bientot il creve, il n'en peut plus.
L'Apoticaire envain lui donne maint distere,
Tous les secours de l'Art deviennent superflus.
Ah, Dit-il, si mourir est un point necessaire,
Pour m'en dedomager, sans faire de facon
Qu'on m'apporte à l'instant le reste du poisson.

An apothecary, protected by an apron, his hat and cane on a chair, and armed with a large clyster syringe advances on the glutton who is being reluctantly dragged from the table, the scene of his feast. The apothecary's assistants with fresh clysters and a commode enter from the right.

PZ. 184

WOODWARD, George Moutard (1760–1809) etched by ROWLANDSON, Thomas (1756–1827)

117 A Cure for lying and a bad memory
[T. Tegg, 111 Cheapside]

Etching hand coloured, cut to 37.50 × 30.00 cm.
Prov.: Purchase
Ref.: George, M. D., 8, 1947, no. 10931

Lettered below design (part):

"A travelling empiric . . . gain'd great credit for his skill in medicine, in fact it was reported that he was capable of curing all diseases . . ."

The scene is the interior of an apothecary's, an alarmed student in cap and gown stands holding his stomach and grimacing. The apothecary stands facing him, his arms in the air and holding a pillbox. His aproned assistant walks away with a sly grin carrying a box "Anti-Fibbibus", the "gilded pill" called "Pillula Memoria". The student complains he has been dosed with Asafoetida, the apothecary declares he is telling the truth and is therefore cured.

PZ. 101

ANON.

118 La Curiosité punie
[n.d. c. 1820]

Etching hand coloured, cut to 18.40 × 23.00 cm.
Prov.: Purchase

A cut-away scene showing both a room interior and the outer corridor beyond a wall and closed door. A smiling maid empties the clyster syringe she was to have applied to her waiting and amused mistress through the door's keyhole and into the eye of a coarse, fat and unwelcome male viewer who recoils in shock.

PZ. 148

MARKS

119 Sham Peter!,
[n.d. c. 1820]
Marks

Etching hand coloured, 20.60 × 12.80 cm. Trimmed to platemark.

Lettered below design:

' – Would it had been done! Thou didst prevent me, I had peopled else this isle with Calibans''

An outrageously fashionable dandy stands admiring himself in a long mirror beside his dressing table, in striped 'Cossack' trousers, boots with long rowled-spurs, and wasp-waisted coat. He says:

"–––––since I cannot prove a lover, I am determined to prove a villain,"

His equally well-dressed young servant in livery brushes his hat. Shelves above the table are full of medicine pots and bottles, including those lettered: "pills from Dr Eady", ("Dr." Eady was a well-known quack whose remedies were much advertised see no. 145.), and "mercury" (an anti-venereal preparation). A book, "The Art of Seduction" lies open on floor near to a clyster syringe.

PZ. 108

FORRESTIER, Alfred Henry "CROWQUILL, Alfred" (1804–1872)
etched by CRUIKSHANK, George (1792–1878)

120 Jealousy. –
Pub^d. November 1st. 1825 by S Knight Sweetings Alley Ryl, X'Change.
A Crowquill Esqr. inv^t.
G Cruikshank fec^t. –

Etching hand coloured, cut to 20.20 × 25.70 cm.
Prov.: Purchase 1956
Ref.: George, M. D., 10, 1952, no. 14905
      Cohn, A. M., 1924, no. 1251

A man sits in deep despair behind a cloth-covered table while small imaginary figures and demons, all alluding to traditional symbols of adultery and cuck-oldry, enact his thoughts: Demons with antlers torment him, a pistol bows and beckons invitingly, a barrister proffers a paper, scene of his hanging, and an elopement of a plump woman with a dashing officer. He clutches his head, his elbow resting on a book "Werter" [J. W. Goethe, *The Sorrows of Young Werther*, 1774], his right fist is on the immediate cause of his troubles, a letter signed "your sincere friend – Anonymous".

As usual, the pictures on the wall continue the theme – "Horn Fair", and Othello smothering Desdemona. Books on table: "The Revenge" [E. Young, 1721], "Don Juan", and "The Cuckoo song book".

PZ. 8, 1–2

[?HEATH, William (1795–1849)]

121 Faith,
Pub^d. Decr. 5th. 1829. by S. Gans Southampton Stret [sic]

Etching hand coloured, cut to 24.20 × 11.70 cm.
Prov.: Purchase

Lettered below design:

"Bolus says that the last thirty doses have done me a World of good! I do'nt [sic] think so myself, but certainly the Doctor must know best."

A thin man standing by an upper window, wearing a tall cap, and a nightgown over shirt, breeches and disordered stockings faces with an anguished expression and addresses the reader as he takes a dose from the spoon in his left hand, medicine bottle in his right.

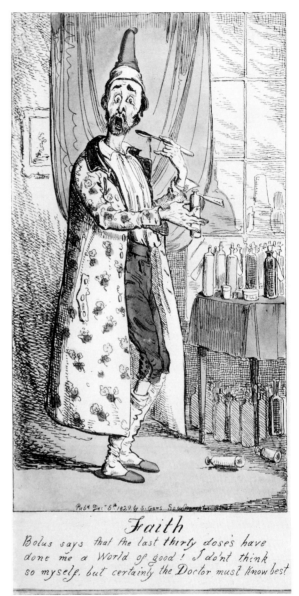

121

A table, and floor beneath it, covered with full and empty medicine bottles and boxes of "PILLS".

PZ. 31

ANON.

122 THE MOST ESTEEMED METHOD OF CURING A FOUL TONGUE according to MODERN PRACTICE!
[n.d. c. 1830]

Lithograph coloured, cut to 39.00 × 31.00 cm.
Prov.: Purchase 1977

Lettered below design:

"Put a Stout Pitch Plaister over the offending <u>Part</u>

when the disorder is at its' height; the effect is certain. — it is also a fine relief for the Ears."

Full length portrait of an unfortunate lady, well dres-

sed and wearing a large trimmed bonnet, vainly waving her arms, her mouth sealed with a pitch plaster.

PZ. 177

POLITICAL AND SOCIAL SUBJECTS

The imagery of pharmacy and medicine is well used in the depiction of general political and social issues portrayed in many caricatures. Of these a proportion are directly relevant to the conflicts taking place among the medical and pharmaceutical worlds, such as those revolving around the restriction of practices (138). But for the majority, medical and pharmaceutical ideas are borrowed to illustrate more general topics such as a scene of political intrigue or a social mood, fashion or event of satirical interest.

The significance of the medical image in relation to the political scene arises primarily from the parallels between the roles of the medical practitioner and politician. Both base their claim to status on an ability to offer specialist advice upon the health, prosperity and welfare of those who seek assistance, a similarity vividly exploited by the artist. Thus, the characteristic functions associated with the medical figure provide a source of graphic imagery, compounded by the ironic comparison which associates the reputation of politicians with the charlatan figure of the medical practitioner. As a result, some of the best known political satires depict an act of medical consultation, which by implication are to be followed by the process of pronouncing a diagnosis, prescribing and administering a treatment.

The majority of these images demonstrate the important role played by the visual reference, immediately recognisable to the audience who viewed these prints (142). To those who were expected to see these prints, an individual could be identified by not only his physiognomy but by the characteristic role they assumed in the scenes that were portrayed. For instance, one of the most frequently repeated visual metaphors of political and social prints of the early 19th century, is that of the nation, symbolised by the long suffering John Bull, being advised by his doctors (136). Other individuals, commonly featured in graphic satire, shown subjecting themselves to the consultation of their medical adviser were equally familiar, especially the figure of George III,

and other politically or socially important characters.

HOGARTH, William (1697–1764)

123 [A Harlot's progress; Plate V]
Plate 5. + W^m. Hogarth inv^t. pinx^t. et sculp^t.

Etching and engraving, cut to 30.10 × 37.30 cm.
WM: – (illegible)
Prov.: Purchase 1966
Ref.: Paulson, R., 1965, no. 125

Third State.

Mary Hackabout sits dying, wrapped in a blanket in a chair by the fireside of her poor lodgings as her two doctors argue violently over whose cure is the superior, and her goods are plundered. The tall thin quack, jumping up from his chair and angrily pointing to his box of pills is most probably Dr. Misaubin (see no. 6, and no. 124), while the seated, portly, self-important, and less excitable quack, who taps a bottle of his medicine with the head of his cane, could be either Dr. Joshua "Spot" Ward (see also no. 5), or Dr. Rock.

Several items of medical interest occur around the room; on the coal scuttle is a spittoon and a paper lettered "Dr Rock" containing some of Mary's teeth (removed as a quack cure for venereal disease). Next to the scuttle is a bed-pan, on the floor nearby is a paper "PRACTICAL SCHEME ANODYNE NECKLACE – ", a current cure for either teething or 'the Secret Disease', while on or over the mantelpiece are medicine bottles, bowls and a bag clyster.

PZ. 186

HOGARTH, William (1697–1764)
engraved by BARON, Bernard. (c. 1700–1762)

124 Marriage A-la-Mode, Plate III
Invented Painted & Published by W^m, Hogarth According to Act of Parliament April 1st. 1745
Engraved by B. Baron

Etching and engraving 38.50 × 46.20 cm.
Prov.: Purchase 1966
Ref.: Paulson, R., 1965, no. 230

Second state.

The quack shown here is probably "Monr. De la Pilule", Dr Misaubin, also satirised in "Harlot's Progress" no. 123 (see also no. 6), and the room or 'museum' was probably in the house of Dr Misaubin, 96 St. Martin's Lane, Westminster. It is full of the various items associated with a virtuoso, or medical man of some education, including anatomical specimens, Egyptian mummies and two peculiar and

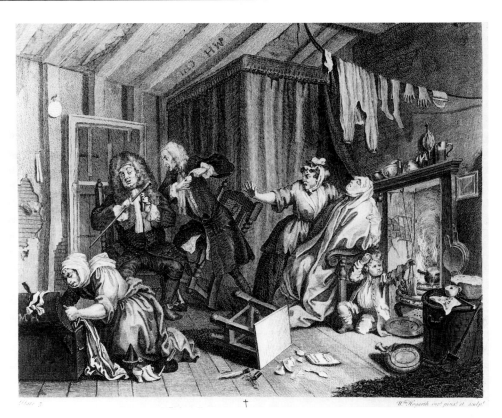

123

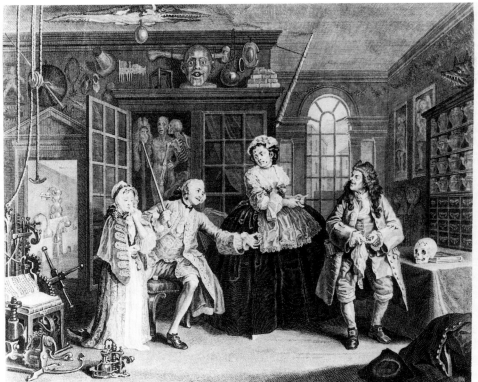

Marriage A-la-Mode. (Plate III)

124

impractical machines of his own design with an explanatory book "–––deux machines superres l'un pour revettre l'epaules l'autre pour servir de tire bouchon inventes par monsr de la pillule vues et approuvees par l'academie royal des sciences–––." However, the narwhal's horn set above the group deftly recalls the barber's pole and the real abilities of the quack.

There are several alternative explanations of this scene, but the nobleman's debauchery and his subsequent contraction of a venereal disease, foreign quacks, a young prostitute and a procuress figure in all. Ireland states it was, 'To show the consequences of his unrestrained wanderings, the author, in this plate, exhibits his hero in the house of one of these needy empyrics, who prey upon public credulity, and vend poisons under the name of drugs.', (Ireland, J., Hogarth Illustrated, 1866, ii, pp. 32–3). The initials "F.C." possibly refer to Fanny Cock, the daughter of an auctioneer 'with whom our artist has had some casual disagreement'.

PZ. 185

MORTIMER, John Hamilton (1741–1779)

125 **Iphigenia's late procession from Kingston to Bristol. ––––– by Chudleigh Meadows.**
Published at Westminst[er] according to Law Ap^l. 15. 1776.
Price 1^{sh}.

Signed on lower margin in ink below design:

_____Then the Duchess was brought into Court attended by her Chaplain, Physician / Apothecary, and three Maids of Honour––––– Morning Post May 16. 1776 – / Dr. Schomberg / Revd. W. Foster. / Duchess Kingston

Etching, cut to 25.00 × 33.90 cm.
Ref.: George, M. D., 5, 1935, no. 5362
      Hein, H., Pharmacy in Caricature, Frankfurt, 1964, no. 9

This satire of a ceremonial procession involving the 'Duchess' Kingston depicts her with the essential members of her household. The lowly apothecary comes last, he is shown as thin, in a 'physical' wig, and a tight coat with deep cuffs. He carries a huge, highly decorated clyster syringe over his right shoulder, his hand on his hip, he wears a dress sword and is possibly a Frenchman. Dr. Schomberg's coat is decorated with hungarian knots and he has a bag-wig and cane. The parson is obese in gown and 'physical', the maids are in open gowns a l'anglaise, with ruched robings and ribbons, with tall piled-high hairstyles and the gauze and feather headdresses popularized by the Duchess of Devonshire. They carry an ominous covered pot, a roll of paper, and a large square "CORDIAL" bottle. The short, fat 'Duchess' is dressed similarly, and swears, "By God an[d]"

PZ. 92

ANON.

126 **Son patriotisme est en Canelle**
Au Coq-Andre, Rue de la grande Tuanderie.
[n.d. c. 1790/92?]

Etching and mezzotint, 20.50 × 12.60 cm.
Rev.: stamp of the "Bibliotheca Lindesiana".

French political satire designed around the image of an apothecary's. Joseph d'André de Bellevue weighs in a set of hand-scales "La Cour" against "Le peuple". On the counter is a pill tile, a hen, and a barrel of "Huile d'Aix". Behind are drug jars and boxes labelled: "ARRETS DU PARLEMENT D'AIX". "Vieilles épices", "Canelle Sucre", "Nouvelles épices", "Alun", "Bonbon au Daupin", "Pastille à la Reine", "Elixir Royal" and "Opium national".

PZ. 56

GILLRAY, James (1756–1815)

127 **LIEUT.GOVERR. GALL-STONE, inspired by ALECTO;___or___The Birth of MINERVA**
'From his head She Sprung, a Goddess Arm'd.' Milton Pub^{sd}. Feby. 15th. 1790. by H. Humphrey No. 18 Old Bond Street
Js. Gillray.
Js. Gillray design, et fect._____

Aquatint hand coloured, cut to 52.50 × 39.20 cm.
WM: WHATMAN
Prov.: Purchase
Ref.: George, M. D., 6, 1938, no. 7721
      Wright, T., The Works of James Gillray the Caricaturist, n.d., London, pp. 116–7

Lettered below design:

"To the opinions of The right hon^{ble}. EDWARD, LORD THURLOW, the EARLS CAMDEN, BUTE, BATHURST, and COVENTRY, George Touchet-BARON-AUDLEY, and PHILIP THICKNESSE Junr. ESQ^r. to the LITERATI, the ROYAL-SOCIETY, the MILITARY, MEDICAL and OBSTETRIC Bodies, this attempt to Elucidate the properties of HONOR and COURAGE, INTELLIGENCE and PHILANTHROPY, is most respectfully submitted, by their humble servant, J^s. Gillray".

Philip Thicknesse (1719–1792), is shown seated and writing at a table. He pauses to listen to Alecto who whispers in his ear, rising from the jaws of hell, and Minerva shoots into the air surrounded by books written by Thicknesse. Other figures in the highly complicated design are Minerva's owl, his monkey Jackoo, or Jocko, which he dressed as a postillion, and Death.

The title arises from Thicknesse's recommendation in his memoirs of laudanum (20, 30, or 40 drops), combined with exercise on a trotting horse to cure gall-stones, he claimed in his memoirs that he was the best of all doctors in England since he had suffered so much himself.

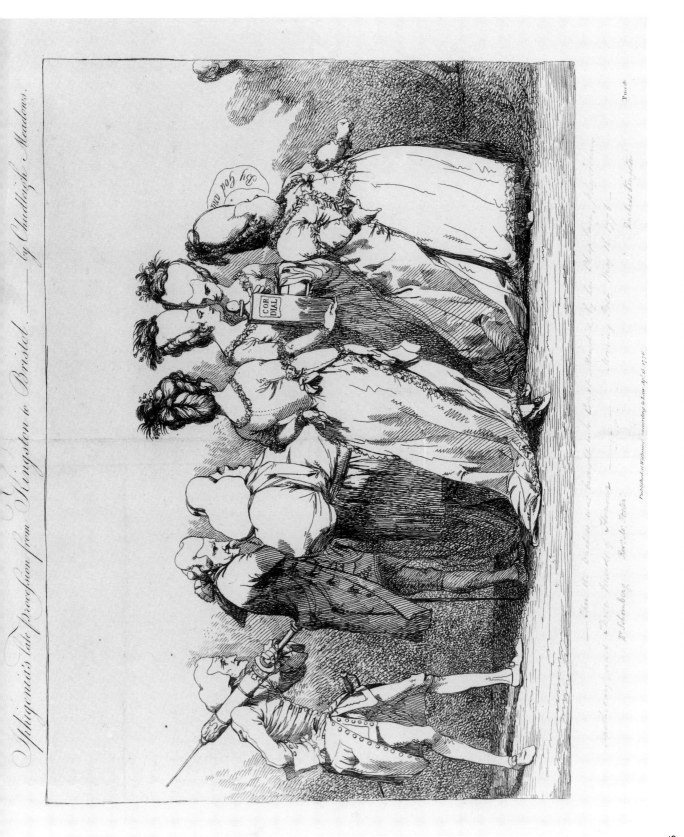

An open book to the left is titled: "Man-Midwifery Analyzed. or a new way to write Bawdy for the instruction of Modest Women With an Emblematic Frontispiece" This, "A ManMidwife touching a Woman", has Thicknesse on his knees before a seated woman, one hand reaching between her legs, the other grasping her bare breast.

PZ. 67

GILLRAY, James (1756–1815)

128 Democratic Leveling; ___ Alliance a la Françoise; ___ or ___ The Union of the Coronet & Clyster-pipe.
Pub^d March 4th. 1796. by H. Humphrey New Bond Street

Etching hand coloured, 36.00 × 25.80 cm.
Prov.: Purchase
Ref.: George, M. D., 7, 1942, no. 8787
   Wright, T., The Works of James Gillray the Caricaturist, n.d., London, p. 201
   Holländer, E., Die Karikatur und Satire in der Medezin, Stuttgart, 1921, pl. 8

Fox and Sheridan are depicted performing the wedding ceremony of Lady Lucy Stanhope and an anthropomorphic apothecary made up of medicinal implements, including a giant clyster, capped with a bonnet-rouge. In reality she married a Mr. Taylor, a surgeon of Sevenoaks, on 26th. March 1796.

Charles 3rd Earl Stanhope, "Citizen" Stanhope, stands on the left, facing in profile to the right, an ardent sansculotte without even breeches, and wearing a bonnet-rouge, guides her towards the breechless bridegroom (Stanhope had taken out a patent for powering ships by steam, hence the miniature 3-masted sailing ship in his coat pocket). Fox wears a surplice and bands and reads from the "Rights of Man", while Sheridan, wearing bands, stands on the right reading from "Thelwals lectures".

On the wall behind them is a picture of a guillotine beheading aristocrats and a heap of coronets, the frame inscribed: "SHRINE OF EQUALITY.".

PZ.62

GILLRAY, James (1756–1815)

129 The DISSOLUTION; or ___ The Alchymist producing an Ætherial Representation.
*Pub^d. May 21st. 1796 by H Humphrey New Bond Street
J^s G^y. des et fec^t.*

Etching hand coloured, 36.90 × 26.00 cm.
Prov.: Purchase 1954
Ref.: George, M. D., 7, 1942, no. 8805
   Wright, T., The Works of James Gillray the Caricaturist, n.d., London, p. 203

This satire attacked Pitt's dissolution of Parliament in 1796, presenting it as a means to distribute patronage to his supporters. Pitt, in royal livery and seated on a "Model of th[e] new Barracks", uses a

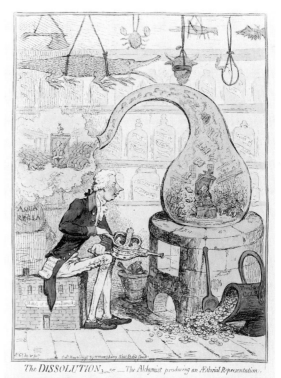

The DISSOLUTION; — or — The Alchymist producing an Ætherial Representation.

129

crown-shaped bellows on a furnace supporting a large alembic containing a scene of the House of Commons, from the spout billows a cloud with an image of Pitt worshipped as a "Perpetual Dictator". By the furnace is a scuttle of "Treasury COLE", which spills gold coins. Various stuffed creatures hang from the ceiling, including a crocodile, a crab, a bull's head, a serpent's egg. The walls of the laboratory are lined with shelves of specie jars labelled: "AQUA REGIA", ,"Oil of Influence", "Extract of British Blood", "Spirit of Sal: Machig[n----]", and "Ointment of Caterpillers". A letter in Pitt's pocket is titled: "Recipe Antidotus Republica".

PZ. 61

GILLRAY, James (1756–1815)

130 Scientific Researches! ___ New Discoveries in PNEUMATICKS! _ or _ an Experimental Lecture on the Powers of Air. ___
520
Pub^d. May, 23". 1802 by H. Humphrey 27 S^t. James's Street ___
J^s. Gillray inv^t. & fec^t –

Etching hand coloured, cut to 38.00 × 47.00 cm.
Prov.: Purchase 1957
Ref.: George, M. D., 8, 1947, no. 9923
   Wright, T., The Works of James Gillray the Caricaturist, n.d., London, p. 289
   Hein, H., Pharmacy in Caricature, 1964, p. 158
   Holländer, E., Die Karikatur und Satire in der Medezin, Stuttgart, 1921, pl. 309

This well known etching is a satire on the fashionable public lectures at the "ROYAL INSTITUTION", and the unfortunate effect of the gas from the pneumatic pump on Sir J. C. Hippisley (1748–1825), whose breeches are almost torn off by the blast. T. Young, the lecturer in chemistry demonstrates assisted by Humphrey Davy (1778–1829), the audience includes: Rumford, D'Israeli, Gower, Stanhope, Pomfret, Englefield, Mrs. Locke, Sotheby, and Denys.

On the demonstration bench, clyster bag, carboys "OXYGEN", "HYDROGEN". Various electrical equipment is visible in a storeroom to the left. A paper on the public bench: "Hints on the nature of Air requir'd for the new French Diving Boat—" refers to the construction of a submarine for Napoleon by the American Robert Fulton.

PZ. 48

ROWLANDSON, Thomas (1756–1827)

131 **Chemical lectures,**
[T. Rowlandson] [1810]

Etching hand coloured, cut to 38.00 × 47.00 cm.
Prov.: Purchase
Ref.: George, M. D., 8, 1947, no. 11605
   Hein, H., Pharmacy in Caricature, Frankfurt, 1964, no. 54

In this accurate depiction of the Surrey Institution, Humphrey Davy lectures to a large and attentive audience. The scowling old man in the back row, in a bag-wig with a paper "Accum's Lectures" (published in 1809 and 1810), in his pocket is a portrait of Friedrich Christian Accum (1769–1838), who was Chemistry Lecturer at the Surrey Institution from 1803.

PZ. 102

GILLRAY, James (1756–1815)

132 **A Pair of POLISHED Gentlemen.**
Publish'd March 10th. 1801, by H. Humphrey, 27 St. James Street.

Etching hand coloured, 35.30 × 25.40 cm.
WM: E & P 1801
Ref.: London & Paris, vii, 1801, p. 77
   George, M. D., 8, 1947, no. 9755

Caricature portraits of two well known dandies. Two round-hatted and cravatted heads issue from the boots of their respective owners, which face each other. They are portraits of Skeffington (in a tassled Hessian) and Martyn Mathew (spurred top-boot). Blacking materials, brushes and bottles are arranged around them with an "Essay on blacking", bottles labelled: "Mr. Broomhills Recipe", "The Princes Recipe", "Spirit of Salt", "PineApple", on a book titled: "CHEMISTRY", a blacking block: "Holdsworth's", and a broken and spilt bottle: "Royal Blacking". In London & Paris, vii, 1801, p. 77,

the good likenesses of the portraits is commented on, as well as the gentlemens' habit of parading up and down St. James's Street in their shining boots.

PZ. 110

GILLRAY, James (1756–1815)

133 **VISITING the SICK**
Pubd. July 28th. 1806. by H. Humphrey. 27. St James's Street.
Js. Gillray fect.

Etching and aquatint hand coloured, 26.20 × 36.20 cm.
WM: J RUSE 1802
Prov.: Purchase 1955
Ref.: George, M. D., 8, 1947, no. 10589
   Wright, T., The Works of James Gillray the Caricaturist, n.d., London, p. 335

A satire on the last illness of Fox, who died in 1806. A group of men and doctors leave the palatial sick room, saying:

"such a day as This! was never seen!"
"O! such a day as This! so renowned so Victorious"
"Well Doctor, have you done his business? – shall we have the Coast clear soon?"
"We'll see!" (he holds bottle of "Composing Draft")

The group around Fox say:

"Ah poor me! I fear my Dancing days are over."
"O Lord! What side can I tack round to Now!"
"I must get back to Ballynahinch! Och! Och!"

Facing him is the Prince: "Alas! poor Charley! – do give him a Brimmer of Sack, 'twill do him more good Abbess, than all the Bishop's nostrums!"

Mrs. Fitzherbert, as an Abbess with a rosary: "Do confess your Sins Charley do take Advice from an Old Abbess & receive Absolution! – here is Bishop O'Bother, 'twill be quite snug amongst Friends you know"

Fox in nightgown and cap with gouty legs sits in a gothick chair, and says: "I abhor all Communion which debars us the comfort of the Cup! – will no one give me a Cordial?"

The Bishop of Meath: "O Tempora, O Mores! – Charley! dear Charley! – remember your poor Soul! – & if you're spared this time give us Emancipation – or!!!"

A whig pamphleteer: "Emancipation! – fudge! – why Dr. O'Bother I thought you knew better!" In pocket a paper: "Scheme for a new Administration"

On the extreme left, Derby comforts a distraught Mrs. Fox: "My dear old Flame Bet, don't despair! – if Charley is pop'd off – a'nt I left to Comfort you?" Bottle at her feet: "TRUE MAIDSTONE"

PZ. 65

ROWLANDSON, Thomas (1756–1827)

134 MORE MISERIES.
page 97.
Pub. April 1st. 1807, by R. Ackerman / Repository of
Arts, 101, Strand.
Rowlandson fecit.

Etching hand coloured, 11.10 × 17.10 cm.
Prov.: Purchase
Ref.: Beresford, J., Miseries of Human Life, 1806
George, M. D., London Life, 1925, pp. 190ff.
George, M. D., 8, 1947, no. 10827

Lettered below design:

"Being pinned up to a door, round the neck, by the
horns of an enraged Over-driven, ox."

Street scene, one of 49 plates based on James
Beresford's work: an ox pins a fat man to the door
of a bow-windowed chemists (bottles outlined in
window), the horns enclosing man's neck. Men with
bludgeons chase the ox, filling the broad street. Two
dogs leap at it, one against the body of an old woman
who falls. Others run away in confusion. A street oil-
lamp standard can be seen in the background.

Bullock-hunting, 'bull-hanking' was a sport of East
London, involving the cutting out of an ox from
Smithfield which would then be chased. Oxen might
also be over-driven by drovers.

PZ. 111

CRUIKSHANK, Isaac (1756–1811)

135 The Porter Brewer and his family – or the Modern
Druggist.
Pub[d] June 8. 1807 by SW Fore (sic) 50 Piccadilly
[Cruikshank I]

Etching hand coloured, cut to 24.00 × 34.00 cm.
WM: A Stace 1801
Prov.: Purchase
Ref.: George, M. D., 8, 1947, no. 10795

Lettered below scene:

"Dedicated to those whom it may concern

A Brewer must brew, and in making of Ale,
When Quassia and Indicus Coculus fail,

Still rather than stop, he'll continue to brew
A Caldron of Mischief to King, Church and you"

The statute K.B. 42 George III c. 33 imposed penalties
on mixing beer with various adulterants, including
quassia, supposedly used instead of hops. The
brewer, wearing a round-brimmed hat and apron,
stands before a large vat of "MODERN INTIRE" into
which he throws "col. narcotic" (a tiny heavy
cavalryman who says: "Here I go neck or nothing").
The brewer motions to the small devils "Tobacco",
"Deadly night shade", "Nux Vomica", "Opium",
"Coculus Indicus", "Hounds Tongue", and "Thorn
Apple" at his feet: "Come along my little boys thats
my Darlings", while two sad putti remark: "Father

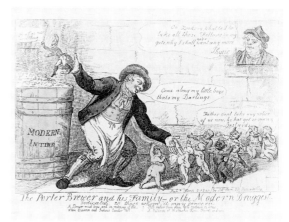

The Porter Brewer and his Family – or the Modern Druggist.

135

dont take any notice of us now, he has got so many
Bastards"

John Bull looks in through a window and says: "Od
lookers, what be I to take all those fellows in my guts,
why I shall ne'er want any more Physic"

PZ. 27

HEATH William (1795–1840)

136 Ministerial Phlebotomy or Bleeding John Bull
Pub 6th of Feb by SWFores 50 Picadilli [sic] [1808]
Folios of Caricatures Lent for the Evening
[Heath W]

Etching hand coloured, cut to 35.40 × 25.40 cm.
Prov.: Purchase
Ref.: George, M. D., 8, 1947, no. 10965

John Bull, stripped to his breeches, his clothes, wig,
and a club "OAK" heaped on the floorboards, flails
his arms in vexed irritation his upper body and head
covered in more than seventeen human-headed
leeches:

"This is Bleeding with A Veangence. If I do not Shake
off Some of these Leaches I shall not have a drop of
Blood Left, why they will never be full & this is the
third set I have had on with in this three years or
so enough to destroy the best <u>Constitution</u>"

Four dying leeches marked "Defaulter 300-000" etc.
lie beneath his upraised right leg by a scroll of "NEW
TAXES". George III looks in from the left margin, and
regards the scene through his spyglass, saying:

"Hard works indeed for poor Johnny. How voraicous
I begin to think they will be too many for him I must
Order some of them off I see".

The semi-literate inscription and affectionate treatment of George III are particularly noticeable here.
Image and text very blurred.

PZ. 190

GILLRAY, James (1756–1815)

137 VERY SLIPPY – WEATHER. _____
_____ *St. James's Street.* _____
London. Published February. 10th. 1808. by H. Humphrey No. 27. St. James's Street.
Etch'd by Js. Gillray.

Etching hand coloured, cut to 25.00 × 19.20 cm.
Prov.: Purchase 1956
Ref.: George, M. D., 8, 1947, no. 11100

A man falls heavily on pavement outside "HUMPHREY No. 27", the publishers. He holds barometer, presumably set for a fall, his wig and hat fall off, coins spill from pocket, and his snuff box falls open. Four men and an urchin with skates under arm look in the bow window of the shop at the prints there, from top to bottom: Taking Physick, a Gentle Emetic, a Brisk Cathartic, Breathing a vein, Charming Well again, In at the Death, French Gingerbd. Bakers, Kick at ye Broad Bottoms, Oh that this so solid Flesh. Two parsons inside the shop look at a caricature of "Catholic Emanci[pation]".

PZ. 53

ANON.
etched by CRUIKSHANK, George (1792–1878)

138 THE COW POX TRAGEDY / – Scene the Last. –
Pub by M Jones 5 Newgate St. //Scourge 1812//
G. Cruikshank Sculpt –

Signed in ink on PZ. 23 below title: "The Sister of the Engraver is a very great Sufferer, having buried [?six] Child[ren]: the [———] [———] folks"

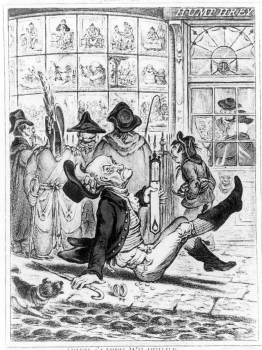

Etching hand coloured, cut to 26.50 × 39.50 cm.
Prov.: Purchase
Ref.: The Scourge, 4, part 20, 1812
George, M. D., 9, 1949, no. 11953
Cohn, A. M., 1924, no. 732
Holländer, E., Die Karikatur und Satire in der Medezin, Stuttgart 1921, p. 357

Lettered below title:

"DEDICATED TO THE ASSOCIATED JENNERAIN COW POXERS OF GLOSTER"

Above a cow slaughtered by Time and a garlanded donkey on an altar "TO THE MEMORY OF/ VACCINA/who died/APRIL the FIRST" between two cornucopiae in the form of scorpions tails, from which spill college reports and roses on the left and various papers marked with the names of diseases, and skulls on the right.

Central scene in the form of a curtained proscenium arch: " 'tis Conscience that makes COW-herds of us all", with two smaller scenes (giving the impression of theatre boxes), on either side, a funeral procession, led by Rowland Hill, issues from a collapsing College of Physicians which falls to rays of "TRUTH", "RELIGION", "REASON", "CANDID INVESTIGATION", and "COMMON SENSE".

PZ. 23
PZ. 24

ROWLANDSON, Thomas (1756–1827)

139 POLITICAL CHEMIST AND GERMAN RETORTS or DISSOLVING THE RHENISH CONFEDERACY.
Pub December 14 1813 by R Ackerman N 101 Strand.

Etching hand coloured, 25.00 × 34.30 cm. Trimmed to platemark.
Prov.: Purchase 1954
Ref.: George, M. D., 9, 1949, no. 12122

A tiny distraught Napoleon, who cries "Oh Spare me till the King of Rome is ripe for mischief yet to come", is partly immersed in a glass alembic over a "GERMAN STOVE", by personifications of the allied nations opposing him, celebrating French setbacks at the hands of the allies. While a Prussian general (?Blucher) puts the lid on the alembic and Bernadotte fills it with "SULPHAT OF SWEDISH IRON", John Bull stokes the fire with coal from "JOHN BULL'S COAL-TUB", a dutchman works the "DUTCH BELLOWS" kneeling beside a pot of "GALL". A Spaniard pounds a mortar marked "SARAGOSSA", on the right of the scene a group, including a Pole, "POLAR STAR" watches a cossack mix a recipe. Receivers from the still are inscribed: "INTRIGUE AND VILLANY", "AMBITION AND FOLLY", "GASCONADE AND LIES", "ARROGANCE AND ATROCITY", "FIRE AND SWORD", "MURDER AND PLUNDER". On the far left is a pile of open books: the title of one "NAPOLEON PROTECTOR OF THE RHENISH CONFEDERACY", erased and replaced by "FRANCIS Emperor of GERMANY restored 1813", "LIBERTY of

VERY SLIPPY WEATHER.

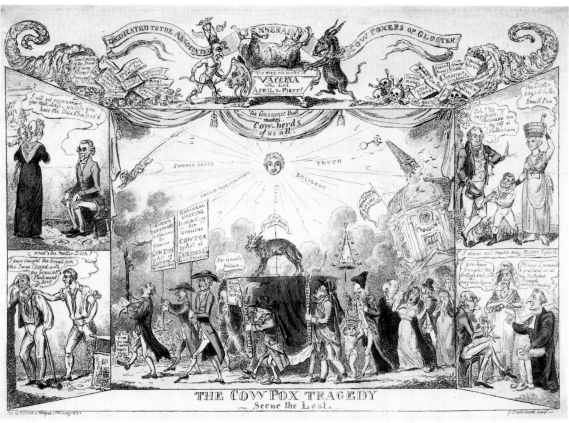

138

CRUIKSHANK, George (1792–1878)

**140 HARD TIMES or, O! Dear what will become of
us! O! dear what shall we do?!!!!!**
311
*Pub^d. Feby. 10th 1814 by T. Tegg Cheapside London
Poor Shanks fect.*

Etching hand coloured, 24.00 × 35.80 cm.
Prov.: Purchase
Ref.: George, M. D., 9, 1949, no. 12185
       Cohn, A. M., 1924, no. 1178

Lettered above the groups:

"Poor Gardeners! Poor Apothecaries! Poor Artists!
Poor Poets! Poor Boney!! Poor Dolley's!!! Jolly
Undertakers –."

During times of hardship it was traditional for the
umemployed to march beneath trade banners to seek
work. Here, following the gardeners are four Apothecaries, under their standard of a mortar on a skull,
One tall and thin, carrying a medicine bottle labelled
"To be well shaken when taken", one short and fat

with a clyster bulging from his pocket. Both are dressed in professional grey, and carry canes, the tops
of which they sniff superciliously. A paper on their
standard: "The Humble Petition of the Poor Apothecaries S[– – –] That they are all starving!!"

On the artists' standard is a palette and brushes with:
"Mr. Wests speech on the gloomy state of the Arts",
and Quill pens lettered: "Rejected MSS". "Poor
Shanks fect" below a self-portrait of Cruikshank.

Bonaparte carries an imperial eagle, with crossed
arms, a tricolour and on top the King of Rome with
huge pigtail.

The prostitutes are grouped below a standard of: an
upturned bottle, torn petticoats and stockings.

The dancing undertakers carry papers: "Bill of mor-
tality", and an (?iron) "PATENT" coffin beneath a
crowned, smiling skull.

PZ. 28

CRUIKSHANK, George (1792–1878)

141 POISONING THE SICK AT JAFFA.
[T Tegg 111 Cheapside] [1814]

Etching and aquatint hand coloured, cut to
24.00 × 30.50 cm.
Prov.: Purchase 1958
Ref.: Combe, W., The Life of Napoleon; a
Hudibrastic poem in Fifteen Cantos by Doctor
Syntax, Edinburgh, 1815, p. 92
George, M. D., 9, 1949, no. 12466
Cohn, A. M., 1924, no. 153

Napoleon in dress uniform, with a big sword, directs
an apothecary in sleeve protectors and apron, holding
a bottle "opium". To the left a mortar and pestle on
stand, carboys and specie jars, hand scales on wall,
and a thermometer in window. A crocodile hanging
above. Sick men in bonnets-rouges are visible in ward
past curtain.

An atrocity satire, based on the story that plagued
French soldiers were given opium on retreat from
Acre, May 1799.

PZ. 26

KING
etched by CRUIKSHANK Isaac Robert
(1789–1856)

142 MILAN COMMISSION!!!_____
Pubᵈ July 1820 by Smolky 18 Rupert Street
I R Cruikshank fecit King sᵗ.

Etching hand coloured, cut to 24.30 × 34.50 cm.
WM: IVY MILL
Prov.: George, M. D., 10, 1952, no. 13763

John Bull a countryman in patched breeches starts
with surprise on seeing a huge leech fastened upon
his back:

"D__me what a monstrous Leech! it not only sucks
blood but honor also!"

"I am not plain Leech, Sir, but by vulgar denomina-
tion. I am called Miss Leech if you please."

Leach, the Vice-Chancellor, in legal dress with bands,
but wearing a large lady's trimmed bonnet, sits on
a corded chest marked COMMISSIO[N] OF—, the
remainder obscured by an open book "Justitia et
honor", he holds a money bag "10 000" in left hand,
and tweaks the ear of a fox, huddled against his knees
which says:

" 'In Law what plea so tainted and corrupt, But,
beings season'd with a gracious voice, Obscures the

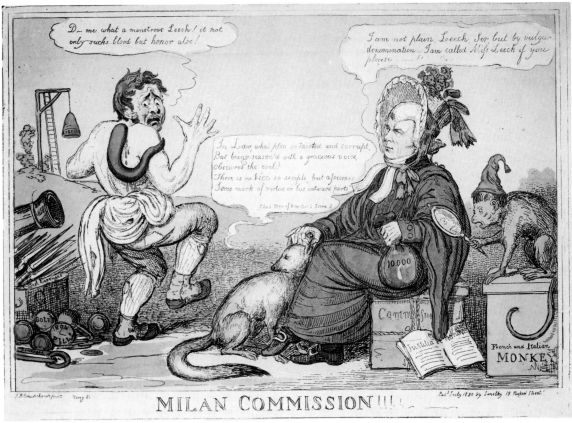

evil ? / There is no Vice so simple, but assumes Some mark of virtue on his outward parts' Shak Mer of Ven. Act3 Scene 2''

Behind Leach a monkey, sitting on a legal document box inscribed ''French and Italian MONKEY[S]'', wearing a combination of fool's cap and bonnet rouge looks into a hand mirror.

Behind John Bull is a heap of weapons, bayonets in a box ''GR''. labelled ''Steel Lozenges'', a quack remedy, cannon balls marked ''BOLUS'' and ''IRON PILLS'', chain shot (used at sea to bring down masts and rigging) inscribed ''Bandages''. On a hill in the distance a cap of ''LIBERTY'' hangs from a gallows.

The Milan Commission was instituted by Leach in 1818 on behalf of the Prince of Wales to go abroad and gather evidence regarding the alleged adultery of the Princess of Wales. This action, though justifiable, outraged public opinion, as the Prince was a notorious adulterer. This satire sees this as one with the general repression of the time.

PZ. 19

ANON.
etched by CRUIKSHANK, George (1792–1878)

143   RADICAL QUACKS giving a New Constitution to John Bull. !
Published by G. Humphrey 27 S^t. James's Street, Feby 4. 1821.
Designed by an Amateur
Etch^d. by G. Cruikshank

Etching hand coloured, 24.60 × 35.80 cm.
Prov.: Purchase
Ref.: George, M. D., 10, 1952, no. 13714
    Cohn, A. M., 1924, no. 1885

''M^r. Bull, you have lived too well, but when we have renovated your Constitution according to our plan the reform will be so complete – ! that you will never again be troubled with any fullness whatsoever !

May be, gentlemen, but you have taken all the honest good blood out of my veins; deprived me of my real supporters & stuck two bad props in their place, & if you go on thus, I shall die before ever my Constitution can be improved.

Never mind M^r. Bull; if we have thought it necessary to take off both your legs you will find the others very good substitutes, this Revolutionary Bolus and docoction of disloyalty, are very harmless but they will restore the general equality of the intestines & remove any obstruction which may prevent us from effecting a Radical Reform in the System.''

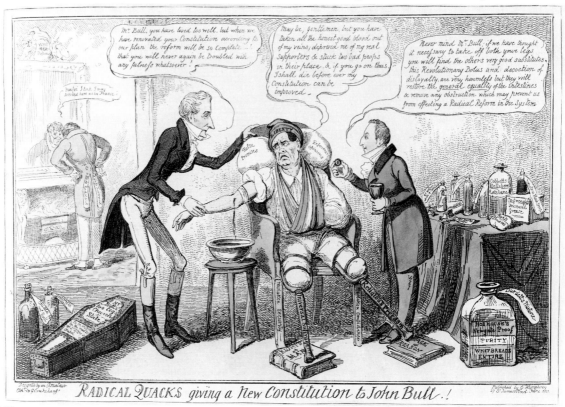

Various issues of 1820 and 1822. John Bull sits in a chair, the legs marked: ''mistaken security'' and ''mistaken confidence'', supported by a pillow of ''False Promises'', and ''Reformers opinions'', between two doctors, Burdett (left) and Hobhouse (right). His legs have been amputated above the knee, the pegs inscribed ''Universal Suffrage'' and ''Religious Freedom'', each rests on a book, ''Rights of Man'' and ''Age of Reason'' by Paine. Legs in coffin ''Mr. Bull's two legs Church & State'', bottles: ''Opiate for Mr. Bull'' ''Sudorific'', behind Burdett who bleeds John Bull wears a cap of ''LIBERTY'', tricolour sling, Bolus and jar of ''Burdett's Mixture''.

''Hobhouse's Newgate Proof, PURITY, WHITBREADS ENTIRE''. Medicines on table: ''Hunts Powders'', ''Cobbetts Hellebore Ratsbane, Hunts Powders Cartwrights Universal Grease, Woolers Black Drops.'' etc.

In background a French dandy bends towards a large mirror: ''Mafoi I tink I may succeed here as in France''. Papers in pockets ''To de Radicaux'' and ''A Messrs Liberaux''. ''Vivit [sic] Rex'' scored through and replaced by ''Populu''. A satire on radical reformers discredited by Cato St. the radicals are associated with the revolutionaries of France and Spain (Liberales connoting Spanish democrats). J.B. victimised by Radical reformers.

PZ. 18

DIGHTON, Richard (1795–1880)

144 One of the Advantages of GAS over OIL.
A LONDON NUISANCE PL^E. 5th.
Pub^d by G. Humphrey 27 St James's Street. LONDON.
Feby. 7. 1822.
Rich^d. Dighton. Inv^t. et Sculp.

Etching hand coloured, cut to 26.70 × 21.80 cm.
Prov.: Purchase
Ref.: George, M. D., 10, 1952, no. 14293

A fashionably dressed woman and a small boy are caught in a gas explosion while walking by a chemists shop, above window and glass door: ''CHYMIST & [DRUGGIST] I = KILLEM''. A carboy strikes her face.

Fragments of window and other objects from the shop fly into the street, including many broken medicine bottles, one: ''LAVENDER WATER . . . BOND ST''. box of ''PILLS'', box of ''LOZENGES'', pens, handscales, pestle and mortar, spatula knife, and two leaflets: ''PERSON'S Electrified on the Shortest Notice'', and ''CURE for DEAFNESS''. The shopman lifts his hands in horror

PZ. 34

CRUIKSHANK, George (1792–1878)

145 Martin's Bill in Operation ---
Published by J. Walker 1824
By George Cruikshank

Etching and aquatint hand coloured, 14.00 × 21.50 cm.
Prov.: Purchase
Ref.: The Family Oracle of Health; or Magazine of Domestic Economy, Medicine and Good Living, 1823–4, pl. to no. VI
George, M. D., 10, 1952, no. 14696

Lettered:

''Martin'', ''Dr. Kitchener'', ''Dr. E---y.''

Three men sit at a table eating oysters while Richard Martin, raids the premises followed by a constable. Walls with shelves of druggists' jars, a mortar and pestle on a box by the door.

Martin's Bill, the first Cruelty to Animals Act, was brought in in 1822. He was well known for bringing actions for cruelty against the poor and then paying the fines himself.

William Kitchiner M.D. (1775?–1827) was an epicure and a writer on cookery. He edited song collections and composed the operetta ''Love among the Roses'' (1822). He sits on a manuscript: ''The Oyster crossed in Love as sung by Messers Sandor & Grimm at Covent Garden   O gentle swain . . .''

'Dr.' Eady was a well-known quack whose remedies were much advertised.

A larder inscribed ''GOOD LIVING'', with food including game, pomegranates, sausages, ''Cherry Bounce'', ''Scots Haggis'', another, the ''LARDER OF DEATH'', has shelves of wet and dry drug jars, shop rounds and bottles, with labels ''OPIUM'', ''Oxalic Acid'', ''Calomel'', and a seed box ''Gamboge''.

PZ. 14

ANON.

146 [Untitled]
[1824]

Etching hand coloured, 32.50 × 41.00 cm.

A street scene with on the left a view inside a ''CHYMIST & DRUGIST'', three shelves of drug jars, carboys and shop rounds. A woman in bonnet and empire dress kneels by boxes marked: ''runaway the 16TH August'', and ''runaway the 19TH of June'' saying: ''alass nothing but Bricks''.

Out in the street are three men, a man in top hat with high stock who says: ''give me my half Part'', with letter under right arm: ''Letters for Prisoners'', and caption ''particular profits'', a fat man in top hat and top boots with five watch fobs ''french Watches'', who says: ''you must wait longer old fellow'', and: ''You look very ill'' to a thin man, bald, short queue, hat under left arm leaning on cane, in Hessian boots, who says: ''am very sick and very poor''. Another plump man, hat under left arm, in top boots: holds in left hand a paper: ''Passport'', and gives a note ''80£'' to fat man.

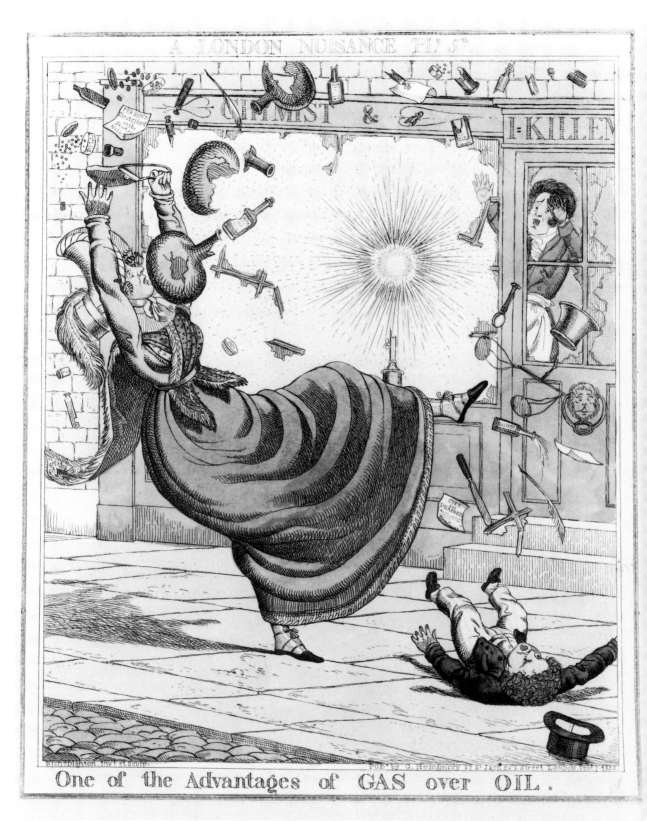

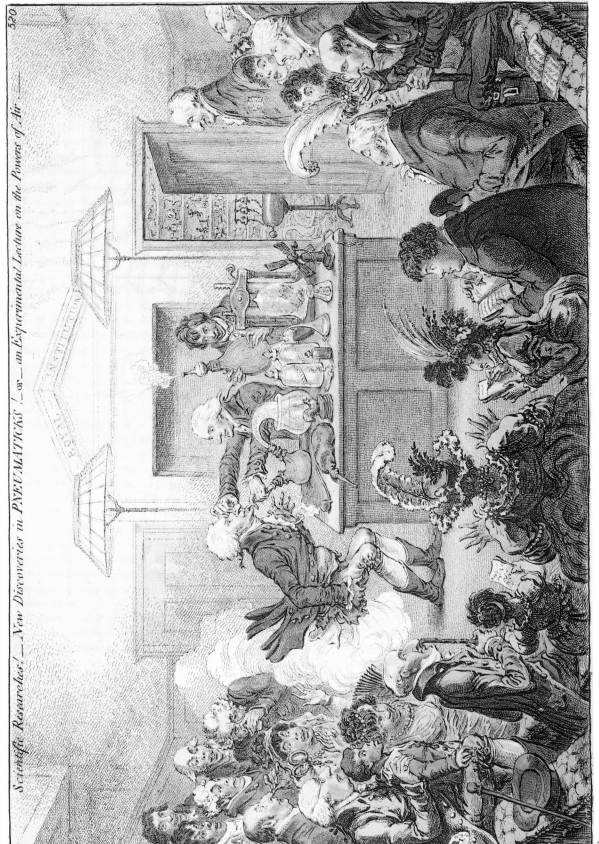

Scientific Researches! — New Discoveries in PNEUMATICKS! — or — an Experimental Lecture on the Powers of Air —

520

130

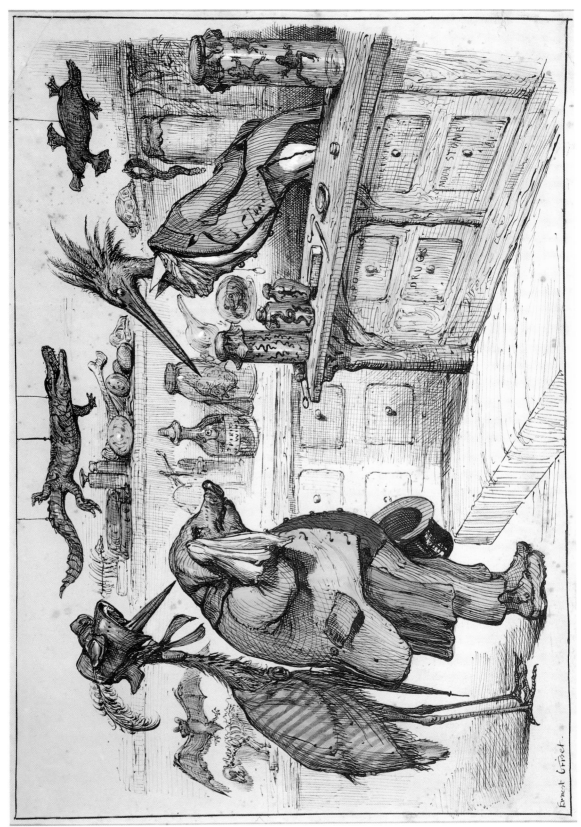

Across the cobbled street are two men with clubs, one in a smock, who chase with a dog a man in Hessian boots captioned above: "executing power and its attributes". The first, with a pistol, says: "It is five minutes past seven".

PZ. 161

HEATH, Henry (fl. 1824–1850)

147 SWEET WILLIAM & GRIZZELL or NEWINGTON-NUNNERY in an Uproar!!!
Pub^d. March. 5th. 1827 – by S W Fores. 41 Piccadilly London.
HH

Etching hand coloured, cut to 21.00 × 32.00 cm.
Prov.: Purchase 1956
Ref.: George, M. D., 10, 1952, no. 15447A

After two prints by Robert Cruikshank (published in February and March 1827) on William Allen's third marriage, set in a Friends' meeting house.

Allen stands facing Grizell, in front of a collection of carboys, seven papers, and graduated measures. She asks: "Is there no hope for me Dear William?", and he replies: "Yes sweet Grizzle I have felt deeply for thee & thou wilt find abundant consolation in the 21st Chapter of Genesis"

Lettered on a book behind the couple:

"No hopes, 'quoth Grizzle as her spouse Looked on her face divine

No hopes quoth he I'm fifty five And thou but sixty nine * When little Isaac first saw light (Translators can't have blundered) His own Mama was Ninty years And his Papa one hundred. Cupid perhaps thou'rt growing old Thy wings may droop, thy head be bald If so thy wounds may now be cold As just a little burn or scald For now behold at fifty five A great & grave divine Led in soft bands as I'm alive By blooming Sixty nine And all do say Love never can Diminish or grow cold She doats upon the very Man He doats upon her Gold

* Aged 72."

The pictures on the wall show Allen and Grizell as Adam and Eve in: "The fall of man", where a rooster cries: "Cock a doodle doo"

On the left is a group of young women, possibly including the five nieces living with Grizell Birkbeck. One falls, saying: "Oh! dear this book has thrown me down and hurt my knee." The book is lettered: "Piety Promoted".

Another swoons, and a helper says: "Send to Plough court for Sal. Volatile" (Allen, first President of the Pharmaceutical Society, had a shop at Plough Court).

Grizell (1758–1837) née Hoare (a banker) married in 1801 William Birkbeck of Norwich (d. 1812).

PZ. 80

CRUIKSHANK, Isaac Robert (1789–1856)

148 RACING   INTELLIGENCE__or__MONEY, MAKES THE MARE TO GO."
Price 1—6__[partly erased]
(Pubd. march 8th. 1827 by R Cruikshank 5 Lownds Terrace Knights Bridge, and [erasure] at 24 [signed in ink] Princess St Licester Square._____
Robert Cruikshank fect.

Etching hand coloured, cut to 33.50 × 39.00 cm.
Prov.: Purchase 1956
Ref.: George, M. D., 10, 1952, no. 15449

A stout Mrs. Birkbeck in bonnet and cloak, long prick spurs on shoes astride a thin grey mare nag races William Allen in Quaker grey, who is a neck ahead on a chestnut. They have almost reached a Friends' MEETING HOUSE, a signpost points to Winchmore Hill. Outside the door are three Quakers two men and one woman:

"Huzza! Huzza! friend William is in for the Plate", "O! Yea!".

Signpost points back "To Wisdom" (reversed lettering), men run after the couple shouting: "Keep the tail up lad", and "Bravo! Bravo!".

These caricatures against Allen said to be from a Quaker source.

"A heat extraordinary will take place on Winchmore Hill, between the favourite high mettled racer Alchemist, and Dr. Syntax's old-mare Grizzle: each carrying feather weight; Alchemist was got by Cooper out of Lady Chab, and has been in training many years, Grizzle was got by Banker out of Quakeress, she has been long noticed for steady paces, never having run a heat for many years. This race has caused great speculation, the winner who is expected to be Alchemist will pocket many thousands by the days sports: he formerly won the – maiden plate against Hamiltonian out of Mary and also the Tottenham purse against Capel out of Hannel Pure. _____"

Allen wrote to a friend in explanation of this marriage; "Should this step appear singular, let it be remembered, that the dispensations through which I have had to pass have been singularly afflictive."

PZ. 9

JONES, T. H.

149 HUMMING ALL THE TRADE IS – OR THE MODERN ALCHEMIST
London. Pubd. march 8. 1827. by G. Humphrey. 27. St James's St.
TJ fect.

Etching hand coloured, cut to 34.75 × 43.00 cm.
Prov.: Purchase 1955
Ref.: George, M. D., 10, 1952, no. 15450

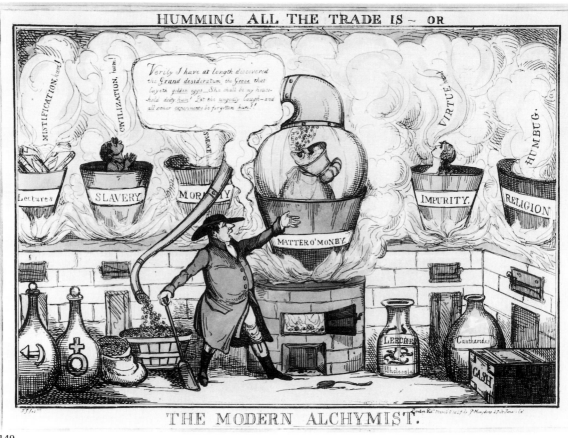

HUMMING ALL THE TRADE IS ~ OR

THE MODERN ALCHYMIST.

149

Another satire on the supposed reasons for William Allen's third marriage. Allen the alchemist in quaker dress, broad-brimmed hat and riding boots, stands spade in hand in his laboratory before a furnace, his left arm thrown out in exultation, he says:

"Verily I have at length discovered the grand desideratum the goose that layeth golden eggs: she shall be my household deity, hum! let the ungodly laugh and all other experiments be forgotten hum!!".

Behind Allen are crucibles containing the personifications of various concepts from which issue captions. The first (from left), containing books marked: "Lectures" and lettered: "MISTIFICATION, hum!", the second crucible: "SLAVERY", from which issues the head of a black slave saying: "CIVILIZATION, hum!", the next crucible is "MORA[LI]TY" from which comes: "SMOKE, hum!", the main central crucible, labelled: "MATTER O'MONEY", with an alembic containing a head of Mrs. Birkbeck, gold coins pour out of her mouth, and fall from the alembic spout into a tub by Allen, the next crucible lettered: "IMPURITY", contains the head of girl from which issues: "VIRTUE, hum!", and finally a crucible of: "RELIGION", from which comes the final comment: "HUMBUG."

Objects heaped around Allen include a carboy: "Cantharides", a box: "CASH", and a jar: "LEECHES Wholesale".

PZ. 87

ANON.

150 A Consultation at the "MEDICAL BOARD"
[n.d.]

Etching hand coloured, 20.00 × 24.80 cm.
Prov.: Purchase

Below a picture titled "PHENOMENA" a portly, well dressed in grey (with jewelled garters), watch etc. doctor sits in a chair facing to the right, he holds an open lancet in his right hand, and motions to his colleague with his left. Beside him, in front of a table with books: "Poetic Emetics by a Knight of the Lancet", "Lessons on Driving by Sir Whip-hand Kt", sits a poodle. On his left is a thin bedraggled man, on his right is a figure composed of medical items, having a mortar and measure for a head, "Lint" for hair, a balance for shoulders, syringe and forceps for arms, drug jars and medicine bottles for legs, pill boxes: "Lozenges" and "Pepper" for feet. It holds a clyster bag and a bottle labelled "Emetic". Around waist a bandage sash holds spatula knives and scissors. Behind him are two bags "L[]ER". A bill headed: "MEG of Wapping at feet of doctor seated above a locked tin marked "TREASURY".

"I am very much obliged to your Honour! I can spare a little blood ____ but spare my flesh for I don't think I have as much as would have satisfied Shylock on my Carcase!"

"I should think my friend you would recomend [sic] him plenty of medicine, and let me bleed him; though he seems poor he's [sic] pay. ——"

"Put on a blister ____ twelve draughts a day ____ sixteen powders ____ a pill every hour ____ a composing mixture ____ a bolus night and morning ____ a proper emetic ____ and then bleed him of Course"

PZ. 145

ANON.

151 **Le Premier Janvier ou les etrennes a Bobonne**
Nº 33,
Genty, Editeur, rue Sᵀ. Jacques, [n.d.]
[-]lami

Lithograph coloured, 21.00 × 20.90 cm.
Prov.: Purchase

[The First of January, or the Housemaid's New Years' Gift]

A dishevelled man carrying an umbrella, feather duster, bellows, broom, tongs, cylster and chamber pot, stands before a seated lady. Curtains in the background.

PZ. 150

ANON.

152 **27, 28, 29 juillet 1830 / 24 Mai 1831, la valeur recompensee.**
[n.d.]
Villain

Lithograph coloured, 20.00 × 28.50 cm.
Prov.: Purchase

Two scenes side by side on a single sheet. The first, subtitled "fermez la Boutique, Voici les rebelles.", depicts the exterior facade in neo-classical style of a "PHARMACIE", the windows shuttered against which a man stands in an act of surrender. A pharmacist emerges from the open door.

The next scene "En Conscience, je ne les ai par gagnee", shows a pharmacy interior, the pharmacist in the uniform of an army officer stands with hand on heart, the other holding a clyster. Behind him is the dispensing counter with box-scales, drug jars and iron mortar and pestle, behind which is a drug run and shelves of shop rounds.

27–29 July 1830 was the uprising leading to Louis-Philippe's accession.

PZ. 152

GRANT, Charles Jameson (fl. 1828–1846)

153 **THE POWER OF ONE, / OR JOHN BULL'S RELAX.**
Pubd. by S Gans, Southampton St.
C J Grant Del.   March 26 1831

Lithograph coloured, 25.40 × 20.50 cm.
Prov.: Purchase

Lettered in a boxed speech bubble:

"My Health and Strength were going Fast
To a Certain Dissolution
When Strange to say One pill at last!
Hath saved my Constitution."

A one-eye-bandaged John Bull, right arm in sling, left leg gouty on cushion, plasters on face, in bedgown, nightcap is seated near a table on which is a box of "GREY'S PILLs" and a bottle labelled "RUSSEL'S PURGE". On the floor lies a paper headed "Reform [Bill]".

PZ. 64

DAUMIER, Honoré (1808–1879)
lithographed by BECQUET

154 **CORTÈGE, du commandant Général des Apothic-aires, le Prince Lancelot de Tricanule à son entrée dans la chambre des pairs**
h-Daumier

Lithograph hand coloured, cut to 48.50 × 61.50 cm.
Prov.: Donation 1951, L'Ordre Nationale des Pharmaciens de France
Ref.: La Caricature, 143, August 1, 1833, pl. 299–300

[Retinue of the Commanding general of Apothecaries, Prince Lancelot de Tricanule, at his entry into the Chamber of Peers.]

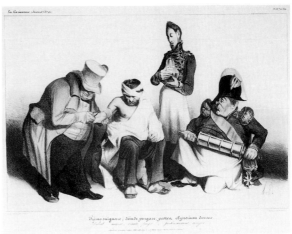

155

Led by a grenadier drummer of the Guard, Lobau, chief of the garde nationale is shown with his signet, the cluster "syringe d'honneur", slung like a sword. Three attendants follow, each carrying an item of regalia on a cushion – a clyster, a seat for a bed-pan, and a ceramic chamber pot (complete with pestle).

The elevation of Lobau to the Peerage on 27 June 1833.

PZ. 32

DAUMIER, Honoré (1808–1879)
lithographed by BECQUET

155   Primo saignare, deinde purgare, postea clysterium donare.
Chez Aubert, galerie véro dodat
h = D.
L. de Becquet rue furstemberg 6.

Lithograph hand coloured, cut to 49.00 × 63.00 cm.
Prov.: Donation 1951, L'Ordre Nationale des Pharmaciens de France
Ref.: La Caricature, 161, December 5, 1833, pl. 337–8

[First to Bleed, Then to Purge, Finally to Give a Clyster].

The scene shows Louis Philippe giving first aid to Wernet the postman run down by the king's carriage. Wernet, with his head bandaged is bled by the king while the Duc d'Orleans stands with a bottle of 'Medicin Leroi', Lobau kneels at the right holding a large clyster at the ready. In this satire the misfortunes of France are symbolised in Wernet's accident.

The caption of French and Latin is derived from Moliere's *Le Malade imaginaire* of 1734.

"D'abord saigner, ensuite purger, posterieurement seringuer/ (Quelques personnes traduisent Deinde par le mot dinde mais c'est un latin de cuisine)".

PZ. 33

DAUMIER, Honoré (1808–1879)

156   LE REMÈDE DE MIMI VÉRON, apothicaire en chef du Constitutionnel
Chez Aubert Pl de la Bourse.
Imp. Aubert & Cie.

Lithograph, 21.00 × 27.00 cm.

Ref.: Le Charivari, May 14, 1850
        Hein, H., Pharmacy in Caricature, Frankfurt, 1964, pp. 160, 167, no. 151

[The Remedy of Mimi Veron, Chief Apothecary of The Constitutionnel] from the series Actualites, no. 124.

"Prenez . . prenez."
["– Take it . . . take it, it is the only thing that can save you!"].

Mimi Veron offers France a large clyster labelled "Solution selon la formule presidence pour dix ans". Veron was the wealthy editor of the newspaper "Le Constitutionnel" which supported Louis Napoleon. He suffered from a neck rash and is always shown with an exaggerated collar and tie.

PZ. 43

HAMILTON, M. D.

157   The Transfusion of blood – a proposed dangerous experiment,
[n.d. c. 1850?]

Lithograph coloured, 33.50 × 41.00 cm.
Prov.: Donation 1981, Lothian-Short, A.

Lettered:

"Doctors (to American workingman) – it may save the patient, but – – if – – a failure you are a dead man;

American workingman – then I won't try it – –"

Bottles marked: "Cobden Tonic", "Mills Bill", "Doc Watterson".

PZ. 160

ANTHROPOMORPHISM

Anthropomorphism, by which animals and inanimate objects are given human form and characteristics, is a device widely used in caricature. First described in G. B. Della Porta's study *De Humane Physiognomia* in 1596, these ideas were followed in the late 17th century by the work of Charles Lebrun and further developed and elaborated in *Physiognomische Fragmente*, by Johann Caspar Lavater, published between 1775 and 1778.

Both subtlety and variety is found in the methods by which anthropomorphism is employed in medical and pharmaceutical images. Some of the most direct caricatures are those which simply substitute animals for humans, adding humour to apparently conventional scenes (160). The comic effect is derived from the incongruous appearance of dumb animals, often adopting human postures, expressions and dress, carrying out recognisable human activities, such as those associated with the doctor or apothecary. Similarly relevant to the medical and pharmaceutical theme are images in which a symbol of medical treatment (characteristically one that inflicts suffering in its application like the clyster, enema or the unpleasant tasting medicine) become, in human form, instruments of retribution or punishment (164). The visual pun forms another important element in the portrayal of the anthropomorphic figure; not only the inevitable monkey performing human tricks, but the doctor or apothecary portrayed as the leech and the quack as the duck.

More complex ideas are conveyed through the anthropomorphic style of Grandville and other French artists of the period. These works develop the use of the animal form to convey through characterisation particular aspects of human folly, weakness and corruption. Grandville, himself, produced a series of cruel and powerful images that focus on the relationship of the innocent patient, the powerless victim of his medical adviser (161). In contrast, typical of the work by Grizet is the affectionate but comic interior view of the rustic shop, in which familiar farmyard creatures take the place of pharmacist and his patients (165).

ANON.

158 Laboratorium mit Affen
[n.d. late 17c]

Engraving, 19.60 × 27.90 cm.

Lettered below design in Latin, French and German:

"Docta etiam sanos Plantis haurite liquores,
Queis aegro medicam sedula praestet opem."

A monkey alchemist and his family work in a laboratory.

PZ. 170

"CP"

159 Guerre aux Libéraux.
Chez Martinet. [n.d. late 18c]
CP.

Etching hand coloured, 31.00 × 41.00 cm.
Prov.: Purchase

In this satire from the French Revolution a file of seven animal-headed figures process from right to left. The first, carrying a halberd, in rich livery says:

"en avant les Débuts? sur l'air: triste raison . . . dans les bienfaits aux Dos."

The next, carrying a candle, bespectacled, and with a drug-jar under his arm:

"le Voila! le G^d. Conservateur ...... des Cornichons."

The third carries a white flag, and plays a clyster syringe:

"moi, j'en détache de la flûte á deux fin; C'est dom-

mage que l'Embouchure n'est pas nete."

There follows a pregnant, dog-headed woman, a loaf of bread under one arm:

"Oh! la la! . . . n'allez donc pas si vite? je sens des débats de droite et de gauche, je vais avoir une Couch de Chiens, c'est le Ventre qui m'annonce ça."

She is followed by a dog-headed man with obstetric forceps and a large knife:

"ne Craignez rien? voila votre Accoucheur."

a cleric follows:

"Bon Dieu! ayez pi pi . . pitié de nous? et jettez des pierre' aux . . des pierres aux autres."

The last figure wears military uniform, a candle-snuffer for a helmet, and pulls a bellows on wheels, to use against the light of liberty:

"avec une Pièce de Campagne comme celle çi, on ne manque jamais de munitions."

PZ.151

MORELL, C. M. B.

160 The Phlebotomist or the Monkey Doctor
[n.d.]

Lithograph coloured, cut to 21.25 × 19.25 cm.
Prov.: Purchase

A scene inside the doctor's room, a monkey wearing cap and gown prepares to bleed his unhappy female patient.

PZ. 93

GRANDVILLE (1803–1847)
lithographed by LANGLUMÉ

161 Les Metamorphoses du jour
N°. 14.
chez Bulla, rue S^t. Jacques, No. 38, et chez Martinet, rue du Coq [n.d]

J. Granville
Lith. de Langlumé

Lithograph hand coloured, 27.50 × 36.00 cm.
Prov.: Purchase

Lettered below design:

"Misere, hypocrisie, convoitise" | "Misery, hypocrisy, covetouness." (sic)

A mouse lies ill in bed while a cat wearing a jacket, waistcoat and trousers stands weeping beside him.

On a table next to the bed is a glass jar of leeches and a bottle labelled 'decine Leroy'. Three crows, one a cleric with a prayer book reading the last rites, one in grey with riding boots, and the other in uniform with a cocked hat and carrying a halberd, stand at the foot of the bed.

PZ. 69

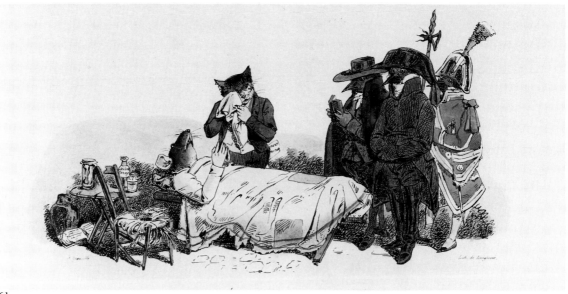

161

GRANDVILLE (1803–1847)
lithographed by LANGLUMÉ

162 Les Metamorphoses du Jour
No. 39.
London 1ˢᵗ, January 1829, Published by Mᶜ.Lean 26,
hay Market
J. Grandville
Lith de Langlumé

Lithograph, 19.75 × 27.25 cm.
Prov.: Purchase
Ref.: Weber, A., Caricature Médicale, Paris, 1936,
        p. 123

"Il y a plenitude nous vous saignerons demain, en
attendant continuer la diete."

"There's redundancy of blood and humours, we'll
bleed you to-morrow, till then, very little food."

Three standing leeches, dressed as doctors in over-
coats, with tophats and canes give their diagnoses to
a cricket, in overcoat and breeches, seated in an armchair, his legs on a footstool. One takes his pulse. On
a small table are bottles, a carafe and a letter.

PZ. 68

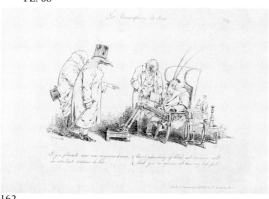

162

GRANDVILLE (1803–1847)
lithographed by LANGLUMÉ

163 Les Metamorphoses du Jour
No 48.
chez Bulla, rue St Jacques, Nᵒ. 38 et chez Martinet, rue
Coq [n.d.]
J Grandville
Lith de Langlumé,

Lithograph coloured, 26.50 × 33.20 cm.
Prov.: Purchase
Ref.: Hein, H., Pharmacy in Caricature, Frankfurt,
        1964, no. 59

"Donnez moi une demi once du metique pour not'
dame qu'est tombee en altaque dans un petit papier;
c'est pas ici une farmacerie."

Mistaking a grocers for a pharmacy a donkey dressed
as a female servant asks a duck, dressed in cap, jacket,
apron and trousers, and pounding a mortar for some
medicine. A kitten dressed as a boy watches.

PZ. 73

CRUIKSHANK, George (1792–1878)

164 Scraps & SKetches Part 3
Designed Etched & Pubᵈ. by George Cruikshank – Febʸ
– 1831 –

Etching hand coloured, cut to 22.50 × 31.50 cm.
WM: J WHATMAN 1830
Ref.: George, M. D., 11, 1954, no. 16851
        Cohn A. M., 1924, no. 180

Collection of visual and verbal puns, part three of
a four part publication, centre design with eight smaller vignettes, the main being a consultation scene
with a doctor made up of a large mortar, his staff a
pestle, medicine bottles for legs and a syrup-jar for
a head sits forward in his chair, in consultation with
his patient, a large pair of bellows, he says:

"Describe the Symptoms"

"Why, you see Doctor—I am upon times so dreadfully puffed up with the wind!—and then again, I have such a sinking in my stomach!"

Books and papers on floor and table: "PNEUMATICS by Professor Blowhard", "The S[trong] Winds do Blow an air adapted to wind instruments by T Blower", "The Art of Puffing", "Mr Bellowshead organ blower Blow Bladder Lane a Treatise on the Blowpipe."

The smaller vignettes depict

(a) A kettle on a grate speaks to a bellows-man: "Well. I suppose you come to blow me up as usual?!!!" He replies: "Sing me a Song then"

(b) Another titled: "Puffing a Grate Singer", the grate sings: "Polly put the Kettle on", And the admirer responds: "O! Bravo! Bravo! Excellent! Beautiful! Divine!!! – Bravo! bravo! Bravissimo!!!"

(c) Bellows dance and sing: "___O! We are the fellows___To sing Old Rose & burn the bellows"

(d) A bellows tinker calls: "any Bellows to mend" ___. A thin compressed bellows says: "ah! I wish you could give me a new pair of lungs!". A female bellows holds out a small bellows-child: "Here master! I wish you would mend my little boy!"

Either side of the main scene are individual figures of a fashionable bellows-woman, with a bonnet, and a guitar player made of a pair of tongs playing a bellows guitar.

PZ. 21

GRISET, Ernest (1844–1907)

165 [The Consultation]
[n.d. c. 1870?]
Signed bottom left: Ernest Griset

Pen and ink with watercolour, 46.00 × 58.00 cm.
Prov.: Purchase 1956

In a rustic pharmacy a lady crane and a boar, dressed as humans stand before a tall pharmacist, also a crane.

PZ. 191

BROWNE, Hablot Knight "PHIZ" (1815–1882)

166 The Blister –
[March 31st 1867]

Pen and ink, 34.00 × 21.50 cm.
Prov.: Purchase

Drawing illustrates a letter (obverse) from the artist which begins "My Dear Sir, Have you become a convert to Homeopathy?" A girl in nightdress looks

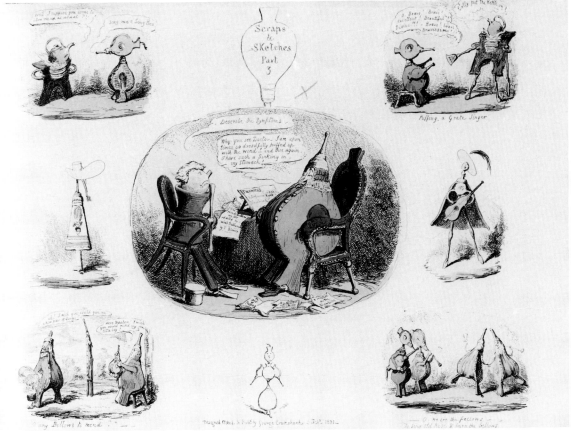

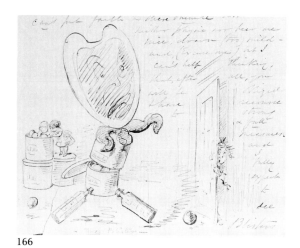

166

around a door to discover a huge, scowling anthropomorphic figure composed of a plaster for the head, leeches for arms, pillboxes for body and medicine bottles for legs. In background two children look into an enormous pillbox.

PZ. 2

BROWNE, Hablot Knight "PHIZ" (1815–1882)

167 [Untitled]
[March 31st 1867]
Signed above design: "and __ Leeches __ arrive in this style! –"

Pen and ink, 34.00 × 21.50 cm.
Prov.: Purchase

Letter (reverse), a huge jar, "The Leeches", containing a mass of writhing leeches surprises woman, chair falls over, her hair stands on end.

PZ. 2. 1

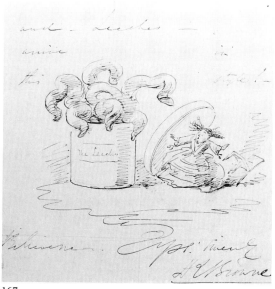

167

ROYAL PHARMACEUTICAL SOCIETY OF GREAT BRITAIN

The majority of the prints within this catalogue belong to the mainstream tradition of caricature undertaken by recognised professional artists. But the fashion for caricature is also reflected in a spirit of amateur interest that found expression among all groups of society. At its most successful, caricature offered scope to communicate issues of universal importance though it could also provide a method to depict ideas of relevance to only a limited audience, informed by a knowledge of particular personalities and issues.

The practice of caricature spread from the satirical journals to a wide variety of publications and periodicals, notably as a form of book illustration and later through the newspaper cartoon. It is not surprising, therefore, that the caricature or comic sketch became a feature of the pages of trade and professional journals, such as the *Pharmaceutical Journal* and the *Chemist and Druggist*. Before the development of successful photograph reproduction, the only graphic illustrations in these journals were those based on original drawings or engravings. Technical diagrams and straight portrait likenesses were most common but the use of comic sketches, usually based on well known pharmaceutical personalities, supplied an increasingly light-hearted and personal character to their pages.

REYNOLDS, Richard Freshfield "Fred" (d. 1907)

168 How the Society might improve the present interesting certificate
[1884]
Signed: R. 84.

Pen and ink with sealing wax, 15.20 × 11.10 cm.

Lettered:

"Pharmaceutical Society of Great Britain"

"We the undersigned do hereby ——— R. F. Reynolds of Leeds is qualified to become a member of above society"

Satire on the design of the Pharmaceutical Society's membership certificate, the supporters, in place of Galen and Avicenna, rendered as an army Major, for the Major Examination, and as a miner, for the Minor Exam.

PZ 122

REYNOLDS, Richard Freshfield "Fred" (d. 1907)

169 The Defender

[1900]

Pen and ink, 20.75 × 13.00 cm.

Ref.: Chemist and Druggist, 57, 1900, p. 810

Text in Chemist and Druggist printed below design:

"DOUGHTY Attfield,
Ever ready,
Draws his pen with
Hand so steady;
Ink, he slings it
By the gallon,
Controverting
Trenchant Allen."

Attfield dressed in uniform as a Boer war Baden-Powell, under a flag "B.P.", for British Pharmacoepeia, advancing and drawing his quill-sword.

John Attfield FRS (1835–1911) studied at the School of Pharmacy where he became Professor of Practical Chemistry in 1862. Founder member of the British Pharmaceutical Conference; founder member of the Institute of Chemistry and elected Fellow of the Royal Society in 1880.

PZ. 115

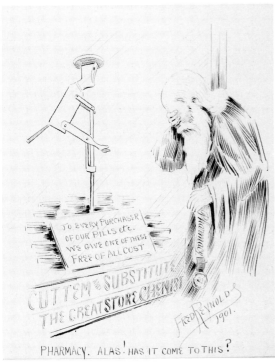

170

REYNOLDS, Richard Freshfield "Fred" (d. 1907)

170 Pharmacy; Alas! has it come to this?

[1901]
Signed: Fred Reynolds

Pen and ink, 20.50 × 16.00 cm.
Prov.: Donation 1901, Reynolds R. F.
Ref.: Chemist and Druggist, 58, 1901, p. 920

Published title: Window-dressing. Copy by the artist, of the original. A pharmacy window display of "CUTTEM AND SUBSTITUTE THE GREAT STORE CHEMIST" showing a pile of pillboxes around a child's wooden toy with a showcard:

"TO EVERY PURCHASER OF OUR PILLS etc. WE GIVE ONE OF THESE FREE OF ALL COST"

Most of Fred Reynolds sketches in the Society's collection were sent as notes or letters to Bremridge and are caricatures of Society subjects which are now unintelligible. However, this is a copy of one of the many Reynolds cartoons published in the Chemist and Druggist between 1886 and 1907. A bearded elderly man holds his head in shame, in his left hand he has the diploma of the Pharmaceutical Society.

A letter to Richard Bremridge, with the drawing explains the subject in some detail, and is worth quoting at length, since it illustrates the conflict between pharmacy as a profession and as a trade:

"Talking the other day to a London traveller who had just worked Lancashire he informed me with great sadness of heart that he had seen in a shop window in Lancashire a man dressed up in coloured linen clothes tearing paper figures out into shapes and handing them to the plebs who came into the so-called pharmacist's shop. He said how awfully ashamed he felt to be connected with pharmacy when the law allowed it to prostitute itself in such a manner. I felt the same and the sketch is the result."

PZ. 113

DOWD, James Henry (1883–1956)

171 [Untitled]

Signed: W. J. V. Woolcock, Secretary and Registrar of the Pharmaceutical Society of Great Britain

Pen and ink, 32.00 × 17.00 cm.
Ref.: The British and Colonial Druggist, 63, 1913, p. 601

Full length portrait of W. J. V. Woolcock, (d. 1947 aged 69) Secretary and Registrar of the Pharmaceutical Society of Great Britain 1913–1918.

PZ. 41

BIOGRAPHICAL NOTES

This index is compiled from the names of artists, engravers, producers and publishers of works in the collection. Where possible names have been identified with appropriate biographical details but otherwise according to the form reproduced on the images, following original spellings and abbreviations.

ACKERMAN (N), Rudolph (1764–1834)
Printer and publisher. His premises at 101 Strand (from 1796–1827), and the periodical he produced were both known as *The Repository of Arts*. Pioneered lithography in this country. Transferred his business to his three younger sons and to his principal assistant, Walton.

ARLAUD, Jacques Antoine (1668–1743)
Artist; portrait painter. Born Geneva, visited London and painted portrait of Queen Caroline 1721.

ATKINSON, John Augustus OWS (c. 1775–c. 1833)
Painter, soft-ground etcher and aquatint engraver. Illustrator of costume, historical and humorous subjects. Travelled abroad and worked in London.

AUBERT Et CIE. (fl. mid. 19th c.)
Family of publishers and engravers. Galerie Vero Dodat, Paris, Place de la Bourse. Known to have published works of Daumier.

BARA, J.
Engraver.

BARON, Bernard (c. 1700–1762)
Engraver. Born Paris instructed by and followed style of Nicolas-Henri Tardieu. Worked in England.

BECQUET
Engraver.

BENNET, J. see SAYER R.
Publisher.

BLACKWOOD, W.
Publisher. Edinburgh.

BOURDEL, Jean Baptiste Desire
Artist.

BRETHERTON, James (fl. 1770–1790)
Etcher and publisher of works of social caricaturists such as Bunbury and James Sayers.

BROCAS, W.
Engraver.

BROOKES, I. B.
Publisher. 9 New Bond St, London.

BROOKE, William Henry (1772–1860)
Illustrator and artist of portraits and figure subjects; exhibited at RA. Nephew of Henry Brooke, the author.

BROWNE, Hablot Knight "PHIZ" (1815–1882)
Humorous artist and illustrator; watercolourist, etcher, lithographer and draughtsman. Worked as illustrator of Victorian novels; succeeded R. Seymour as Dicken's illustrator in 1836.

BULLA
Publisher. 38 Rue St Jacques, Martinet, Rue Coq.

BUNBURY, Henry William (1750–1811)
Amateur caricaturist, a prolific producer of gentle, non-political, satires towards the end of 18th century, usually etched by others. Equerry to the Duke of York.

"C"
Engraver.

COLE, William (fl. 1765–1792)
Engraver and printer. 109 opp. Warwick Lane, Newgate Street 1784–92.

COOK, Thomas (1744–1818)
Engraver of caricatures, portraits and decorative subjects influenced by his contemporaries and known for his copies of Hogarth's prints.

COOK, I.
Publisher. Paternoster Row, London.

COURCELL, A.
Illustrator, engraver and draughtsman. Monogram "CP"

CROWQUILL, Alfred see FORRESTIER, Alfred Henry

CRUIKSHANK, George, Snr. (1792–1878)
Caricaturist and polemicist on temperance; draughtsman and etcher. Second son of Isaac Cruikshank, and younger brother of Isaac Robert. Originally worked for his father but from his death in 1810 concentrated on political and social satire, following and replacing J. Gillray as principal artist for Mrs Humphrey's. From late 1840s increasingly involved in work for the temperance movement.

CRUIKSHANK, Isaac Robert (1789–1856)
Caricaturist, miniature painter and illustrator; painter and etcher. Eldest son of Isaac Cruikshank and brother of George to whose style his work has been compared. Early career in merchant navy before becoming an artist and satirist. Great success with illustrations for E. Pierce's *Life in London* but died in poverty.

CRUIKSHANK, Isaac (1756–1811)
Caricaturist, genre painter, illustrator, draughtsman; painter and etcher. Born in Edinburgh, father of George and Isaac Robert.

"CW"
Engraver.

DAGLEY, Richard (c. 1765–1841)
Engraver. Worked in London, his early career spent working for a jeweller and watchmaker.

DARL(E)Y, Matthew (active c. 1754–81)
Caricaturist, paper-hanging manufacturer, engraver and printseller, 39 Strand (from 1767–80). Artist's colourman and teacher. Produced over 300 caricatures and dominated period between Hogarth and the early works of Rowlandson and Gillray. Concentrated on social subjects after 1766, mainly from works of amateurs and his pupils and produced vols. of *Macaronies, Characters and Caricatures*.

DARL(E)Y, Mary (active c. 1756–77)
Print-seller, etcher and teacher of caricature and etching. For some prints signed "M. Darly" there is uncertainty over their attribution between Mary or her husband and partner, Matthew.

DAUMIER, Honoré (1808–1879)
Lithographer, painter, sculptor. Born Marseille, one of the best known satiric artists of his time, who worked for Charles Philipon, publisher of *La Caricature* and *La Charivari*. Produced some 4,000 political caricatures and satirical scenes of Parisian life. Served 3 months in prison, with the Editor of *La Caricature*, for a satire on Louis-Philippe.

DAVISON, Thomas
Publisher. 11 Paternoster Row, London.

DAVISON, William (1781–1858)
Publisher, printer, chemist and druggist of Alnwick.

DELPECH, Francois-Seraphin (1778–1825)
Engraver and lithographer, portraitist after contemporary works.

DIGHTON, Richard (1795–1880)
London caricaturist; etcher and draughtsman. Son and successor of Robert Dighton (q.v.), between 1814–28 producing small, full-length, profile portraits in the "Dighton Style".

DIGHTON, Robert (1752–1814)
Engraver, printseller, drawing master and caricaturist. Published caricatures of his contemporaries 1792–1812. Earned notoriety for his theft of Rembrandt etchings from British Museum but was pardoned when they were returned in 1806. 12 Charing Cross 1794–99.

DOWD, James Henry (1883–1956)
Painter, dry-point etcher. Regular contributor to *Punch* from 1906.

DOYLE, John "H.B." (1797–1868)
Irish caricaturist, lithographer and portrait artist. Studied under Italian landscape painter, Gabrielli, and miniaturist, W. Comerford. Best known for "H.B." sketches, produced between 1829–1851.

DUCOTES, A.
Lithographer. 10 St Martins Lane.

DUNTHORNE, J.
Artist.

EGERTON, W.
Publisher and author. London

ELMES, William "XYZ" (fl. early 19th c.)
Caricaturist, etcher and draughtsman, in the style of G. Cruikshank. Possibly the same artist as line, stipple and aquatint engraver working in late 18th c.

ENGELBRECHT, Martin (1684–1756)
Printseller and engraver. Born Augsburg, brother of Christian. Engraved plates after Rugendas and other masters, produced illustrations of Ovid's *Metamorphoses*.

FAIRBURN, John (active 1812–32)
Chart, map and printseller. 2 Broadway, Blackfriars 1812–21; 13 Broadway 1822–32.

FILLOEUL
Publisher and engraver. Rue du Fouarre.

FORES, Samuel William (fl. 1786–1841)
Printseller, bookseller and engraver. Produced many prints of caricatures imitating Gillray and others. Premises known as "Caracture Warehouse": 50 Piccadilly 1795–1820; 41 (sometimes 40) Piccadilly 1822–1841.

FORRESTIER, Alfred Henry "CROWQUILL A"
(1804–1872)
Caricaturist, illustrator, writer and comic artist. Worked

on newly founded *Punch* and in early career he drew social satires that were engraved by G. Cruikshank. Later career devoted to children's book illustration.

FRESCHI, A.
Engraver.

GANS, S.
Publisher. Southampton St, London.

GENTY, Charles (b. 1876)
Publisher and collaborator on satirical journals. 33 Rue St Jacques.

GERARD, Jean-Ignac Isidore "GRANDVILLE" (1803–1847)
Best known by his pseudonym "Grandville". Caricaturist, draughtsman, watercolourist and lithographer. Though born in Nancy, France, where he worked successfully as a lithographer and for *La Caricature*, specialising in anthropomorphic representations, his works were also widely bought and popular in England.

"G L S"
Artist.

GILLRAY, James (1756–1815)
Caricaturist; etcher, draughtsman, aquatint and stipple engraver, after his own and amateurs' designs. Trained under classical engravers, W. W. Ryland and F. Bartolozzi and at RA Schools. Early works published by Robert Wilkinson of Cornhill, S. W., Fores and finally Mrs Humphrey. Regarded as the first professional caricaturist in this country, his work covering a wide range of political and social subjects. His last print appeared in 1811 and he died insane.

GIRALDON-BOVINET
Publisher. 5 Rue Pavée, St Andrée.

GRANDVILLE, see GERARD, Jean-Ignac Isidore

GRANT, Charles Jameson (fl. 2nd quarter 19th c.)
Caricaturist and draughtsman; wood engraver, lithographer and etcher. Leading artist of penny Radical papers.

GRISET, Ernest (1844–1907)
Illustrator and draughtsman. Born Boulogne-sur-Mer and studied under Louis Gallait and came to London in 1860s. Known for his animal drawings, demonstrating their human qualities, with a view similar to the work of Grandville. Worked for *Fun* and *Punch*.

"G W"
Engraver.

HAMILTON, M. D.
Artist.

HAUTECOEUR MARTINET
Publisher. Rue Du Coq, Paris.

HEATH, Henry (fl. 1824–1850)
Caricaturist; draughtsman, lithographer and etcher. Worked after his own designs and imitator of styles of John Doyle "HB" (signed "HH") for Messrs Fores, Cruikshank and Seymour. Employed by the publisher, Spooner, to produce political caricatures. Possibly brother of W. Heath.

HEATH, William "Paul Pry" (1795–1840)
Watercolourist and caricaturist; etcher, draughtsman, lithographer. Military painter. Produced the first caricature magazine in Europe, *The Glasgow*, later *Northern Looking Glass* 1825–26. His popularity as a caricaturist was eclipsed by the humorous work of J. Doyle and R. Seymour after 1834.

HODGSON, Orlando (active c. 1823–44)
Printer from established family of printers. 111 Fleet Street, 1836–44.

HOGARTH, William (1697–1764)
Painter and best known engraver of 18th c. Played a major part in the development of graphic social satire, though scorned the "modern fashion, caricature" for distorting all aspects of physiognomy (particularly the anthropmorphic representation of man to animal) rather than concentrating on the more subtle transformation of facial detail, at which he excelled. Apprenticed to silverplate engraver, Elias Gamble. As a result of the piracy of his own work, he agitated for the enactment of the Engravers' Copyright Act 1735.

HOLLAND, William (active c. 1782–1803)
Proprietor of print and caricature warehouse. 50 Oxford Street 1782–1803. Imprisoned for one year and fined £100 for selling Paines's *Letter to the Addresses* 16 Feb. 1793.

HUMPHREY, Hannah (fl. 1778–1830)
Trading as Hannah Humphrey 1778–1807; as Henry Humphrey 1811–1817; as George Humphrey 1820–1830. Exclusive publisher of Gillray's cartoons from c. 1791 but only surpassed rivals, Fores and Holland, after move to St James's Street: At St Martin's Lane 1778; 18 New Bond Street 1778–82; 51 New Bond Street 1783–89; 18 Old Bond Street 1790–94; 37 New Bond Street 1794–97; 27 St James's Street 1797–1824; 24 St James's Street 1826–1830.

HUMPHREY, William (active c. 1764–88)
Engraver and printseller, mainly of portraits. Supplier to major collectors. 227 Strand, 1772–c. 1788.

JEAN
Publisher. St Jean de Beauvais, Paris.

JOHNSON, C. (active c. 1793–4)
Printseller and publisher of *Wonderful Magazine* 1793–4. Succeeded by Alex. Hogg.

JONES, Maurice (active c. 1801–1817)
Printer; 5 Newgate Street 1809–17, previously at 1 Paternoster Row.

JONES, T. H.
Engraver.

KENDRICK, J.
Publisher. 54 Leicester Square, London.

KING
Artist.

KNIGHT, S.
Publisher. Sweetings Alley, Royal Exchange, London.

LAGUILLERMIE, Frederick Auguste (b. 1841 fl. 1863–1923)
French painter, illustrator and etcher of portraits and genre subjects, after British 18th c. his British and French contemporaries and Old Masters.

LANGLUMÉ
Engraver and lithographer.

LEFEVRE & KOHLER (fl. 1893)
Publishers, engravers and printers. 52 Newman St. Previously L. M. Lefevre of Newman Street.

LEMERCIER
Engraver. Rue de Seine, Paris.

LISLE, Joe
Caricaturist.

LONGMAN, HURST, REES, ORME (active 18th c. to present)
Trading name of booksellers and publishers of 39 Ship and Black Swan, Paternoster Row from 1826–1850. One of London's largest publishers around 1800, acquired many valuable provincial businesses.

LOUTHERBOURG, Phillippe Jacques de, RA (1740–1812)
Caricaturist, landscape painter, illustrator, inventor, mystic and quack. Born in Strasbourg, studied under F. G. Casanova and Carlo Vanloo. Worked in England from 1771, particularly concentrating between 1775–80 on caricature. Friend of Gillray and influenced by Mesmer, Cagliostro, and especially by Richard Brothers, he came to believe himself a prophet capable of healing others without medicine.

MAISON BASSET
Publisher. 33 Rue de Seine, Paris.

MANSERGH, R. St G. (active c. 1770–78; d. 1797)
Amateur caricaturist.

MARKS & SONS (mid 19th c.)
Printer. Houndsditch, London 1859.

MARRYAT, Capt. Frederick RN CB FRS (1792–1848)
Novelist, amateur caricaturist and draughtsman. Grandson of Thomas Marryat M.D. Served at sea and visited St Helena, and North America. Some of his caricactures were said to have hindered his advancement in the navy.

MARTINET
Publisher.

MAURON
Caricaturist.

MCLEAN, Thomas (active c. 1822–38)
Printer of fine art and publisher. 26 Haymarket 1822–1865.

MILLER, John
Publisher. London Bridge St.

MONNIER, Henri (1805–1877)
Notable French caricaturist. Worked for Charles Philipon's La Caricature, later Le Charivani.

MORELL, C. M. B.
Caricaturist.

MORTIMER, John Hamilton RA (1741–1777)
Painter, etcher, draughtsmen of portraits and dramatic subjects. Studied under J. Reynolds.

NAU, J. (fl. mid. 20th c.)
Caricaturist.

NEWTON, Richard (1777–1798)
Caricaturist and miniaturist; aquatint engraver, etcher and draughtsman. Prolific caricaturist during his short working life, in the manner of his contemporaries, particularly Gillray.

NOËL, F.
Engraver.

NOËL, Leon
Caricaturist.

NOYER, A.
Publisher. Paris.

ORME, Edward (active c. 1801–1823)
Printseller in ordinary and engraver to the King. New Bond Street, 1803–23; 59 New Bond Street 1801–1817.

PATERRE
Caricaturist.

PIGAL, Edme Jean (1798–1872)
French satiric artist and lithographer, known for genre subjects.

POND, Arthur (1705–56)
Caricaturist and portraitist; printer, etcher and line engraver after his own and his contemporaries designs. Work includes prints after Italian caricatures and Italian Masters and he was important in promoting knowledge of Italian caricature in England.

PRY, Paul see HEATH, William

RAINAUD
Artist and engraver.

REEVE & JONES
Publisher. 7 Vere St, London.

REYNOLDS, Richard Freshfield "Fred" (active c. 1884–1905; d. 1907)
Amateur artist, pharmacist. Cartoons on pharmaceutical subjects published in the *Chemist and Druggist*. Director of Reynolds and Branson Ltd, Leeds. Son of Richard, one of the founders of the British Pharmaceutical Conference.

ROWLANDSON, Thomas (1756–1827) Caricaturist, illustrator, watercolourist, draughtsman; etcher and aquatint engraver. Educated at RA Schools, and travelled abroad extensively on the Continent. Major figure in the history of satirical art, particularly social caricatures. Lived and worked in London for publishers, including S. W. Fores, R. Ackerman and T. Tegg.

SALA, George Augustus Henry (1818–1896)
Illustrator, author and journalist. Worked as theatrical scene painter before becoming a book illustrator. Correspondent for the *Illustrated London News* and *The Daily Telegraph*.

SAYER, R. (d. 1794; active c. 1745–94)
Print, map and chartseller. In business as R. Sayer & J. Bennett 1774–84. Sayer re-issued Darly's *Macaronie* series. One of the main print publishers of the period, great rival of Bowles. 53 Golden Buck, Fleet Street 1745–94.

SEYMOUR, Robert "SHORTSHANKS"
(c. 1799/1800–1836)
Caricaturist, illustrator and draughtsman; lithographer and etcher. Worked as a comic illustrator and caricaturist though is best known as first illustrator of Dickens' *Pickwick Papers*. Acquired his signature-name as a reference to Cruikshank's, on whose work he attempted to model his own.

SHARPE, A.
Publisher. London.

SHERINGHAM, J.
Caricaturist.

SHERWOOD, NEELY, JONES
Publisher. Paternoster Row, London.

SHORTSHANKS see SEYMOUR, R.

SIDEBOTHAM, I.
Publisher. 24 Lowr Sackville St, Dublin.

SMOLKY
Publisher. 18 Rupert St.

SNEYD, Rev. John (1766–1835)
Amateur caricaturist. Friend and patron of Gillray and was Rector of Elford for more than 40 years.

SPOONER W.
Publisher. 377 Strand, London.

STYPULKOWSKI
Engraver and artist.

TEGG, Thomas (c. 1776–1846)
Printer, bookseller, stationer and paper dealer. A famous populariser who published over 4,000 works. Trading as Thomas Tegg 1805–32; as T. Tegg and Son 1834–38; as T. Tegg 1839–46. 111 Cheapside 1805–32 and 73 Cheapside 1824–46.

TEMPEST, Pierce (1653–1717)
Printseller, publisher and possible mezzotint engraver of portraits after his contemporaries.

TOMLINSON
Publisher. 24 Great Newport St, London.

TORRE, Anthony (fl. 1767-late 1780s)
Printseller and publisher of satires 1781–2. Sister-in-law married Paul Colnaghi to whom he gave up his London business. Son of Giovanni Battista, printseller.

TREGEAR, G. S.
Publisher. Various addresses in Cheapside; 96 Cheapside and 123 Cheapside, London.

VILLAIN, Gerard Renard (fl. c. 1760)
French engraver of portraits after other artists.

WALKER J(ohn?) (mid 18th c.)
London printseller and carver.

WARREN
Publisher. Old Bond St, Whittaker, Ave Maria Lane.

WATTEAU, Jean-Antoine (1684–1721)
Major artist; painter and draughtsman. Born Valenciennes, son of a plumber, in early life drew grotesques.

"W E"
Engraver.

WEST, T.
Caricaturist.

WIGSTEAD, Henry (d. 1793)
Caricaturist and etcher. Friend of Rowlandson and etched some of his designs.

WOODWARD, George Moutard (Murgatroyd), (c. 1760–1809)
Caricaturist and watercolourist. Between 1794–1800 produced political caricatures, some in original "strip" form. His work was often etched by Rowlandson, Gillray, Roberts, Williams and I. Cruikshank.

"XYZ" see ELMES, W.

SELECT BIBLIOGRAPHY

The works cited in this bibliography are a selection of those consulted in the preparation of this catalogue. To assist the user, it has been divided into sections relating to the major categories of reference works and is intended as both a guide to the sources used in compiling this work and to further study.

Given the wide scope of secondary material available, this bibliography is deliberately selective. The major works cited here should provide additional information concerning more specialist sources, in particular monographs, catalogues and studies on individual artists.

General Works on Caricature

Atherton, H. M., *Political Prints in the Age of Hogarth. A Study of the Ideographic Representation of Politics*, Oxford, OUP, 1974

Cohn, A. M., *George Cruikshank. A Catalogue Raisonné of the Work executed during the Years, 1806–77*, London, The Bookman's Journal, 1924

Duffy, M., (Gen. Ed.), *The English Satirical Print 1600–1832*, 7 vols., Cambridge, Chadwyck Healy, 1986

Everitt, G., *English Caricaturists and Graphic Humourists of the Nineteenth Century*, London, Swann Sonnenschein, Le Bas & Lowery, 1886

Feaver, W. and Gould, A., *Masters of Caricature: from Hogarth to Scarfe and Levine*, London, Weidenfeld and Nicholson, 1981

George, M. D., *From Hogarth to Cruikshank: Social Change in Graphic Satire*, London, Viking, 1967

George, M. D., *English Political Caricature. A Study of Opinion and Propaganda*, 2 vols., Oxford, Clarendon Press, 1959

Gombrich, E. H., and Kris E., *Caricature*, London, Penguin, 1940

Jouve, M., *L'Age D'Or De La Caricature Anglaise*, Paris, Presses De La Foundation Nationale Des Sciences Politiques, 1983

Lambourne, L., *An Introduction to Caricature*, London, HMSO, 1983

Paulson, R., *Hogarth's Graphic Works: First Complete Edition*, New Haven, Conn., Yale University Press, 1965

Reid, G. W., *Descriptive Catalogue of the Works of George Cruikshank*, 3 vols., London, Bell & Daldy, 1871

Stephens, F. G., and George, M. D., *Catalogue of Political and Personal Satires. . . . in the British Museum to 1832*, 12 vols, London, British Museum, 1870–1954

Victoria and Albert Museum, *English Caricature. 1620 to the Present*, London, Victoria and Albert Museum, 1984

Wright, T., *The Works of James Gillray the Caricaturist*, London, Chatto and Windus, n.d.

Medicine and Pharmacy in Caricature, including Anthologies and Catalogues

Boussel, P., *Histoire Illustrée de la Pharmacie*, Paris, Guy Le Prat, 1949

Boyer, P. E., *In Sickness and in Health. Medicine and Health Care in 19th-Century French Prints, A Salute to the New Jersey Pharmaceutical Industry*, New Brunswick, New Jersey, The State University of Jersey, Rutgers, 1984

Cabanès, Dr. , *La Médecine en Caricature*, 4 vols., Paris, P. Longuet, 1925–1928

Gee, E. S., and Haupt, S. M., *Selections from the Clements C. Fry Collection of Medical Prints and Drawings, in Exhibition in Yale University on the Occasion of the Sesquicentennial Celebration of the School of Medicine*, New Haven, Conn., Yale University, 1960

Hein, W.-H., *Die Pharmazie in der Karikatur*, Frankfurt am Main, Govi-Verlag, 1964

Helfand, W. H., *Drugs and Pharmacy in Prints (An Exhibition of Prints and Drawings from the Collection of William H. Helfand)*, Toronto, 1967

Helfand, W. H., James Morison and his pills. A study of the nineteenth century pharmaceutical industry (inc. Caricatures on James Morison and Morison's Pills: A Check List), *Trans of the Brit. Soc. for the Hist. of Pharm.*, 1974, 1, (3), 102

Helfand, W. H., John Bull and his Doctors, *Veröffentlichungen der Internationalen Gesellschaft für Geschichte der Pharmazie*, 1966, **28**, 131

Helfand, W. H., The medical theme in American political prints, *Imprint*, 1980, **5**, (1), 2

Helfand, W. H., *Medicine and Pharmacy in American political prints (1765–1870)*, Madison, Wisconsin, American Institute of the History of Pharmacy, 1978

Helfand, W. H., Pharmaceutical and Medical Valentines, *Pharmacy in History*, 1978, **20**, 101

Helfand, W. H., Medicine and Pharmacy in British political prints – the example of Lord Sidmouth, *Med. Hist.*, 1985, **29**, 375

Helfand, W. H., Medicine and Pharmacy in French political prints, *Pharm. in Hist.*, 1975, **17**, 119

Helfand, W. H., and Julien, P., *Medicine and Pharmacy in French political prints. The Franco-Prussian War and the Commune*, in Acta Congressus Internationalis Historiae Pharmaciae Bremae, MCMLXXV

Helfand, W. H., and Julien, P., *La Pharmacie par L'Image (Exposition organisée a l'occasion du Congrès International d'Histoire de la Pharmacie, Paris 1973)*, Paris, Société d'Histoire de la Pharmacie, 1973

Helfand, W. H., and Rocchietta, S., *Medicina e Farmacia nelle caricature politiche Italiane 1848–1914*, Rome, Edizioni Scientifiche Internazionali, 1982

Holländer, E., *Die Karikatur und Satire in der Medizin*, Stuttgart, Verlag von Ferdinand enke, 1921

Julien, P., and Helfand, W. H., La caricature medico-pharmaceutique comme arme politique, in *Acta Congressus Internationalis XXIV Historiae Artis Medicinae*, 2 vols., Budapest, Museum, Bibliotheca et Archivum Historiae Artis Medicinae De. I. Ph. Semmelweis Nominata, 1976

Lothian-Short, A., Englische Pharmazeutische Karikaturen, *Zur Geschichte der Pharmazie*, 1961, **13**, 1

Lothian-Short, A., Pharmaceutical Caricatures, in *Die Vortrage d. Hauptversammlung in Dubrovnik 1959, Stuttgart, Veröffentlichungen d. Intern. Gesellschaft f. Geschichte d. Pharmazie*, 1960, 89–96

Tait, H. P., Medicine and Pharmacy in Caricature, *Pharm. Journ.*, 1963, **190**, 247

Vogt, H., *Medizinische Karikaturen von 1800 bis zur Gegenwart*, Munich, J. F. Lehmann verlag, 1960

Weber, A., *Tableau de la Caricature Médicale*, Paris, Editions Hippocrate, 1936

Wittop Konig, D. A., *Geneeskunde en farmacie in de Nederlandse politieke prent 1632–1932*, Haarlem, Netherlands, Merck Sharp & Dohme, 1979

Zigrosser, C., *Ars Medica (A Collection of Medical Prints Presented to the Philadelphia Museum of Art)*, The Philadephia Museum of Art, Philadelphia, 1955

Zigrosser, C., *Medicine and the Artist (137 Great Prints)*, 3rd ed., New York, Dover, 1970

Historical Background

Bynum, W. F., and Porter, R., (Ed.), *Medical Fringe & Medical Orthodoxy 1750–1850*, London, Croom Helm, 1987

Jameson, E., *The Natural History of Quackery*, London, Michael Joseph, 1961

Loudon, I., *Medical Care and the General Practitioner 1750–1850*, Oxford, Clarendon Press, 1986

Maple, E., *Magic, Medicine and Quackery*, London, Robert Hale, 1968

Matthews, L. G., *History of Pharmacy in Britain*, London, E. & S. Livingstone Ltd., 1962

Porter, R., and Porter, D., *In Sickness and in Health. The British Experience 1650–1850*, London, Fourth Estate, 1988

Thompson, C. J. S., *The Quacks of Old London*, London, Brentano's Ltd, 1928

Waddington, I., *The Medical Profession in the Industrial Revolution*, Dublin, Gill and Macmillan Ltd., 1984

Woodward, J., and Richards D., (Ed.), *Health Care and Popular Medicine in Nineteenth Century England*, London, Croom Helm, 1977

General Reference Works

Bénézit, E., *Dictionnaire critique et documentaire des Peintres, Sculpteurs, Dessinateurs et Graveurs*, Paris, Libraire Grund, 1976

Brown, P. A. H., *London Publishers & Printers c. 1800–1870*, London, British Library Reference Div., 1982

Chubb, T., *The Printed Maps in Atlases of Great Britain and Ireland 1579–1870*, London, Homeland Association, 1927

Griffiths, A., *Prints and Printmaking*, London, British Museum Publications, 1980

Hind, A. M., *A Short History of Engraving & Etching*, London, Constable, 1908

Houfe, S., *The Dictionary of British Book Illustrators and Caricaturists, 1800–1914*, Woodbridge, Suffolk, Antique Book Collector's Club, 1978

Mackenzie, I., *British Prints. Dictionary and Price Guide*, Woodbridge, Suffolk, Antique Book Collector's Club, 1987

Maxted, I., *The London Book Trades 1775–1800*, Folkestone, Kent, Dawson & Sons, Ltd., 1977

Riberio, A., *A Visual History of Costume. The Eighteenth Century*, London, Batsford, 1983

Todd, W. B., *A Directory of Printers & Others in Allied Trades 1800–1840*, London, Printing Historical Society, 1972

Williams, G. C., *Bryan's Dictionary of Painters and Engravers*, Port Washington, Kennikat Press, 1964

INDEXES

TITLE INDEX